# MCQs in Clinical Pharmacology

# MCQs in Clinical Pharmacology

**Bleddyn Davies** PhD MRCP
Department of Geriatric Medicine,
St Tydfil's Hospital, Merthyr Tydfil

**Alan Sinclair** BSc MRCP
Department of Geriatric Medicine,
University of Birmingham

**Stephen Jackson** MD MRCP
Department of Clinical Pharmacology,
St Bartholemew's Hospital, London

**Churchill Livingstone** 🏛
EDINBURGH LONDON MELBOURNE AND NEW YORK 1989

CHURCHILL LIVINGSTONE
Medical Division of Longman Group UK Limited

Distributed in the United States of America by Churchill
Livingstone Inc., 1560 Broadway, New York, N.Y. 10036,
and by associated companies, branches and
representatives throughout the world.

First published 1989
Reprinted 1991

ISBN 0-443-03729-9

**British Library Cataloguing in Publication Data**
Davies, Bleddyn
 MCQs in clinical pharmacology.— (Multiple choice
questions).
 1. Pharmacology — Questions & answers
 I. Title  II. Sinclair, Alan  III. Jackson, Stephen
 615'.1'076

**Library of Congress Cataloging in Publication Data**
Davies, Bleddyn, MD
 MCQs in clinical pharmacology.

 (Multiple choice questions)
 1. Pharmacology — Examinations, questions, etc.
I. Sinclair, Alan.  II. Jackson,
Stephen.  III. Title.  IV. Series.  [DNLM.
1. Pharmacology, Clinical — examination
questions.  QV 18 D255]
RM301.13.D38  1988  615'.1'076  88-6117

Produced by Longman Singapore Publishers (Pte) Ltd
Printed in Singapore

# Preface

Multiple choice questions (MCQ) are an anathema to many but are essential components of qualifying and postgraduate examinations, hence our idea of putting together this book. We have used MCQ as a way of revising with students large therapeutic areas in a short time. This was done by the students trying the MCQ and then discussing the answers afterwards. Our aim is for the book to be used in this sort of way, i.e., to learn from as well as practice at MCQ. Most exams have moderately severe questions plus a few really hard ones to sort out honours candidates and this is the way the papers have been structured. Some MCQ in the book, in each paper, are hard so that the book (we hope) will be useful to undergraduates and doctors studying for the MRCP. Nearly all of the questions have been based upon patients we have seen and they are of a management nature thus showing that clinical pharmacology is not a dry "academic" subject but of enormous every-day use for all doctors! If the reader has any suggestions or criticisms (even destructive ones) the authors would be very grateful to know them, please address any to IBD (St Tydfil's Hospital, Merthyr Tydfil). We would like to thank Professor Paul Turner, BSc, MD, FRCP of St. Bartholomew's Hospital, London, Professor Peter Sever MA, PhD, FRCP and Professor Sir Stanley Peart MD, FRCP, FRS of St. Mary's Hospital, London for their enthusiasm and teaching which has given us the inspiration for this small but difficult to write book.

1989

IBD
AJS
SHDJ

# Chapter 1

**1.1 Digoxin**

    **A** is preferred to ouabain in sudden onset rapid atrial fibrillation because its action is more rapid

    **B** prolongs the refractory period of the bundle of His by direct action and augmenting vagal tone

    **C** is the treatment of choice for congestive heart failure

    **D** may cause multiple ventricular ectopic beats

    **E** directly increases atrial muscle refractory period

**1.2 Lignocaine**

    **A** may cause bradycardia by augmenting vagal tone

    **B** slows the heart by producing beta-adrenoceptor blockade

    **C** may cause hypotension

    **D** lowers the threshold of patients for convulsions

    **E** is effective in treatment of ventricular arrhythmias

**1.3 Jaundice due to cholestasis may occur**

    **A** with phenelzine treatment of depression

    **B** in chronic paracetamol therapy

    **C** long-term treatment of acne vulgaris with tetracycline

    **D** the use of depot phenothiazines to treat schizophrenia

    **E** as a side-effect of oral contraceptives

**1.4 Simultaneous use of the following pairs of drugs is in general contraindicated**

    **A** amitriptyline and amphetamine for withdrawn depression

    **B** treatment of hypertension with debrisoquine in a patient receiving imipramine for depression

    **C** metoclopramide and aldactide (combined spironolactone and hydroflumethiazide)

    **D** phenylbutazone and warfarin

    **E** aspirin and phenobarbitone

1.1   A **False**   ouabain given intravenously is quicker in action
      B **True**    main action on SA node is via vagus but direct action
                    on AV node and bundle increases refractory period
                    and may rarely cause heart block
      C **False**   diuretics are treatment of choice. Digoxin is a
                    positive inotrope but its use in sinus rhythm is
                    controversial
      D **True**    by increasing automaticity in conducting tissue and
                    myocardium; supraventricular arrhythmias are
                    commoner
      E **False**   digoxin shortens action potential of myocardium
                    (remember digoxin shortens the e.c.g. QT interval)

1.2   A **False**
      B **False**   no influence on any adrenoceptors
      C **True**    higher plasma concentrations after higher doses or
                    patients with heart failure (less liver blood flow and
                    less clearance of lignocaine) may cause myocardial
                    depression
      D **True**    paraesthesiae, drowsiness, dissociation are other
                    neurological side-effects
      E **True**    (easy) — along with mexilitene, tocainide, flecainide,
                    phenytoin, procainamide, quinidine, amiodarone

1.3   A **False**   monoamine oxidase inhibitors can cause acute
                    hepatic necrosis rather than pure cholestasis (were
                    you fooled?)
      B **False**   only after liver failure in overdosage
      C **False**   only relationship of tetracyclines with bile is
                    excretion therein (so useful in infective cholangitis)
      D **True**    all phenothiazines may cause cholestatic jaundice
      E **True**    due to 17-α-alkyl nortestosterone derivatives
                    (progestagens) in combined pills. Other 'liver effects'
                    of oral contraceptives: hepatic adenomas, Budd-
                    Chiari syndrome. (Hons level this)

1.4   A **False**   nonsense. Amitriptyline is a 'sedative' tricyclic (cf.
                    desipramine — more stimulant), amphetamine
                    stimulates but is addictive — use only in narcolepsy
                    and child hyperkinetic syndrome
      B **True**    antagonism beloved of clinical pharmacologists:
                    imipramine blocks debrisoquine uptake into
                    sympathetic neurons where debrisoquine blocks
                    neurotransmission. Adrenergic neurone blockers are
                    less used now
      C **False**   no known contraindication
      D **True**    phenylbutazone potentiates warfarin (displaces it
                    from plasma proteins)
      E **False**

**1.5   Cutaneous infections with *Candida albicans* may be treated with**

  A   in severe cases with systemic nystatin therapy
  B   amphotericin B cream
  C   oral griseofulvin for at least 6 weeks
  D   miconazole cream
  E   metronidazole ointment

**1.6   Gentamicin**

  A   is mainly metabolised in the liver, undergoing 90% biliary excretion with very little drug entering the urine
  B   is well absorbed orally
  C   in severe pyelorephitis can, with advantage, be combined with a loop diuretic to increase entry of gentamicin into the kidney
  D   can produce permanent vestibular nerve damage
  E   is used most effectively when plasma concentrations of the drug are measured

**1.7   Synthetic derivatives of oestradiol**

  A   may cause deep vein thrombosis
  B   can be used to produce remission in postmenopausal breast carcinoma
  C   are drugs of choice to suppress lactation in the puerperium
  D   are a rare cause of the Budd-Chiari syndrome (hepatic vein thrombosis)
  E   can cause orofacial dyskinesias

**1.8   The use of oral contraceptives may be unwise or totally contraindicated in**

  A   severely obese females who smoke
  B   severe spasmodic (primary) dysmenorrhoea
  C   with a past history of migraine
  D   in patients receiving simultaneous phenytoin for treatment of epilepsy
  E   in patients with recently cured depression

1.5  A **False**    nystatin is too insoluble for parenteral use but can be given orally or topically. Amphotericin B is used parenterally for systemic (not cutaneous) candidiasis

    B **True**     ointment also available

    C **False**    griseofulvin only of use for dermatophytic fungi, candida is a yeast

    D **True**

    E **False**    metronidazole only active against anaerobic bacteria and protozoa (trichomoniasis, amoebiasis)

1.6  A **False**    obvious — it is good for severe pyelonephitis because large amounts enter urine

    B **False**

    C **False**    this combination increases nephrotoxicity (similarly for loop diuretics given simultaneously with cephaloridine)

    D **True**     also for deafness (like other aminoglycosides, e.g. streptomycin)

    E **True**     measurement of trough and peak levels is mandatory in severe illness or renal impairment

1.7  A **True**     for all oestrogens

    B **True**     cf. 'oestrogen-dependant', premenopausal carcinoma

    C **False**    lactation may cease spontaneously but bromocriptine is drug of choice. Oestrogens work but risk thrombo-embolic effects

    D **True**

    E **False**    only direct c.n.s. effects is chorea

1.8  A **True**     increased risk of thrombosis and impaired glucose tolerance

    B **False**    oral contraceptive is alternative treatment to a non-steroidal anti-inflammatory drug

    C **True**     oral contraceptives may exacerbate migraine

    D **False**    — as worded (badly). Phenytoin induces liver hydroxylases which increases metabolism of oral contraceptives, however a 50 $\mu$g oestrogen pill probably provides safe contraception

    E **True**     oral contraceptives may produce/exacerbate depression. This may be averted by pyridoxine supplements, hence the marketing of combined contraceptive pill/pyridoxine packs (without good evidence to support their use)

**1.9    Nitrazepam, A 1,5-benzodiazepine**

A    is a powerful inducer of liver microsomal hydroxylase
     enzymes
B    is a more powerful hypnotic than diazepam
C    must be used cautiously in elderly insomniacs who may be
     more sensitive to benzodiazepines than the young
D    is the drug of choice to control alcohol withdrawal
E    prolonged use of this drug can cause tachyphylaxis

**1.10    Desferrioxamine**

A    is a useful adjunctive drug in treatment of lead poisoning
B    can be used to treat thalassaemia
C    is well absorbed orally but is metabolised in the liver with
     loss of activity due to biliary excretion and enterohepatic
     circulation
D    in acute use can cause a distal myopathy
E    is an indirect acting sympathomimetic like tyramine

**1.11    Calsynar® (salmon calcitonin)**

A    is better absorbed orally than from intramuscular injection
     sites because of inflammatory reactions caused at injection
     sites
B    is of great use to treat hypocalcaemia
C    is a good prophylactic to prevent pain occurring in Paget's
     disease of bone
D    if given to patients with Paget's disease of bone can
     alleviate painful symptoms
E    is a safe alternative to use of cholecalciferal in osteomalacia

**1.12    Intravenous dextrans**

A    are contraindicated in treatment of shock following long-
     bone fractures
B    invalidate blood cross-matching
C    can result in renal toxicity in patients with pre-existing renal
     failure
D    Decrease incidence of fat embolism if given pre- and
     perioperatively in hip replacement and repairs of femoral
     shaft fractures
E    can be used to provide calories in total parenteral nutrition

**1.13    Chloramphenicol therapy is**

A    usually indicated in meningococcal meningitis
B    the treatment of choice for typhoid fever
C    sometimes associated with optic neuritis
D    effective in *Haemophilus influenzae* meningitis
E    dangerous in renal failure

1.9 A **False**  do not confuse with barbiturates which are
    B **False**  they have equal efficacy
    C **True**   increased somnolence, confusion, accidents and
                 enuresis may result from ignorance of this
    D **False**  chlormethiazole (Heminevrin) probably best in
                 Britain, chlordiazepoxide is used in USA
    E **True**   tolerance to sedative and anticonvulsant effects of
                 benzodiazepines is well-known

1.10 A **False**  dimercaprol or penicillamine chelate lead
     B **True**   desferrioxamine may prevent Fe overload in β-
                  thalassaemia major, where frequent blood
                  transfusions are needed
     C **False**  is not absorbed orally so can be given orally in Fe
                  overdose to prevent Fe absorption
     D **False**
     E **False**  rubbish this

1.11 A **False**  calcitonin a peptide is obviously not stable by mouth
     B **False**  calcitonin lowers blood calcium
     C **False**  tricky! Pain is the indication for use of calcitonin in
                  Paget's disease, but calcitonin is not given
                  prophylactically
     D **True**   a diphosphonate can also be used to treat pain
     E **False**  rubbish. Calcitonin has no effect on gastrointestinal
                  calcium absorption and is not used in osteomalacia

1.12 A **False**  may be useful in reducing venous thrombosis
     B **True**   plasma expansion with dextrans can be of use in
                  shock but blood must first be taken for cross
                  matching. Haemaccel is a new alternative to dextrans
     C **True**   take care!
     D **False**
     E **False**  dextrans cannot be metabolised to provide a supply
                  of glucose

1.13 A **False**  drug of choice is benzylpenicillin
     B **True**   cotrimoxazole or mecillinam are of use
     C **False**  chloroquine, clioquinol (enteriovioform) and tobacco
                  smoking are the only drugs to cause optic nerve
                  damage, phenothiazines crossing the placenta
                  damage the developing uveal tract. Quinine too in
                  overdose causes optic neuritis
     D **True**
     E **True**   excretion is mainly urinary: lower dose in renal
                  failure

**1.14  Cloxacillin**

 A   is indicated in all staphylococcal infections
 B   is useful for β-lacto mase-producing cocci
 C   is absorbed after oral administration
 D   is rapidly excreted in urine
 E   is of major use in haemolytic streptococcal infections

**1.15  Griseofulvin**

 A   is effective for treatment of ringworm
 B   can be used to treat *Candida albicans* infections
 C   is well absorbed after a fatty meal
 D   is contraindicated in patients with liver disease
 E   is effective for treatment of *Malazessia furfur*

**1.16  In treatment of severe diabetic ketoacidosis in adults**

 A   intravenous sodium bicarbonate should be given
     immediately to correct acidosis
 B   two litres of intravenous fluid are needed in the first 90–120
     minutes
 C   oxygen therapy may be required
 D   the amount of insulin which is required is related to the
     initial blood glucose concentration
 E   infusion of potassium is rarely needed

**1.17  Patients with acute intermittent porphyria should not be given**

 A   oral contraceptives
 B   chlorpromazine
 C   sulphonamides
 D   penicillins
 E   glucose

1.14  A **False**    only in penicillinase-producing ones
      B **True**     bad Q — if you knew A, you knew this too!
      C **True**     absorption is poor so flucloxacillin is preferred for
                     oral use
      D **True**     all penicillins are well excreted in the urine
      E **False**    phenoxymethylpenicillin (penicillin V) (oral) or
                     benzylpenicillin (penicillin G) are drugs of choice

1.15  A **True**
      B **False**    griseofulvin is only effective against fungi, candida is
                     a yeast
      C **True**     unlike many drugs which are absorbed less well after
                     food
      C **True**     griseofulvin can cause deterioration of liver function
      E **False**    *M. furfur* causes tinea (pityriasis) versicolor:
                     Whitfield's ointment or clotrimazole (Canesten)
                     cream are used topically

1.16  A **False**    acid-base imbalance will usually be corrected after
                     insulin, electrolyte and fluid replacement.
                     Bicarbonate should only be given in severe acidosis
      B **True**     osmotic diuresis from glucose and vomiting induce
                     large fluid loss
      C **True**     any acidotic state favours anaerobic metabolism,
                     oxygen aids reinstatement of aerobic glucose
                     oxidation
      D **False**    only small intravenous or intramuscular doses of
                     insulin are needed, this is especially true in non-
                     ketotic hyperosmolar diabetic coma
      E **False**    potassium replacement is always needed

1.17  A **True**     oestrogens induce synthesis of aminolevulinic acid
                     synthetase, a rate-limiting enzyme in porphyrin
                     production, so leading to overproduction in
                     genetically susceptible individuals. Any other
                     diseases exacerbated or precipitated by oral
                     contraceptives? — Yes, hypertension, acne, vulgaris,
                     migraine, depression
      B **False**    chlorpromazine is a good drug for sedating such
                     patients
      C **True**     sulphonamides may be given when patients
                     complain of red urine in the mistaken belief that a
                     urinary tract infection is present
      D **False**    penicillins are safe
      E **False**    intravenous glucose infusions repress synthesis of
                     aminolevulinic acid synthetase ('glucose effect') and
                     are used to treat acute attacks (intravenous haematin
                     has a similar effect) (well done if you got this one!)

**1.18   Phenytoin**
  A   may produce ataxia
  B   can cause cholestatic jaundice
  C   can cause lymphadenopathy
  D   myopathy is a common side-effect
  E   macrocytosis may occur with prolonged therapy

**1.19   Increased excretion of uric acid in urine occurs with**
  A   chlorothiazide
  B   allopurinol
  C   sulphinpyrazone
  D   colchicine
  E   phenylbutazone treatment

**1.20   Cimetidine**
  A   inhibits gastric acid secretion by antagonizing activity of $H_2$-receptors
  B   has a long terminal elimination half-life and so can be given infrequently
  C   is an antagonist at androgen receptors
  D   its effect is enhanced by cigarette smoking
  E   may cause hypochlorhydria with intestinalization of gastric epithelium

1.18 A **True**    in overdosage cerebellar signs occur; acute
                   confusion and peripheral neuropathy may also be
                   caused by phenytoin
     B **False**
     C **True**    primidone and para-aminosalicylic acid (PAS) also
                   cause this ('pseudolymphoma' reaction)
     D **False**   commoner drug causes of myopathy are
                   corticosteroids (especially triamcinolone) and
                   potassium depletion
     E **True**    phenytoin and phenobarbitone may produce folate
                   deficiency with macrocytosis in blood and
                   megaloblast in bone marrow

1.19 A **False**   the reverse thiazides compete with uric acid for
                   tubular secretion
     B **False**   allopurinol, a xanthine oxidase inhibitor decreases
                   rate of urate production
     C **True**    sulphinpyrazone also an 'antiplatelet' drug
     D **False**   careful. Colchicine is useful in acute gout because of
                   its anti-inflammatory action preventing lysozomal
                   enzyme release
     E **True**    metabolites are uricosuric and sodium retaining

1.20 A **True**    competitive, reversible, inhibition
     B **False**   it has a relatively short half life and is often given
                   four times daily, although twice daily use can heal
                   ulcers and recent work shows once a day dose may
                   work
     C **True**    can cause gynaecomastia and impotence
     D **False**   cigarette smoking antagonizes action of cimetidine
     E **True**    observations in animals led to concern about this in
                   man and possible links with bacterial overgrowth,
                   nitrosamine formation (carcingens) and gastric
                   carcinoma.

# Chapter 2

## 2.1 In pulmonary tuberculosis

A in Great Britain intramuscular streptomycin daily for 6 months is the treatment of choice
B para-aminosalicylic acid must be included in the first 2 months treatment
C any treatment regimen must contain isoniazid
D the Mantoux test result may be negative if the infection is very severe
E 9 months is a sufficient duration of treatment if 3 antituberculous drugs are combined for the first 2 months of treatment

## 2.2 Increased incidence of ampicillin rash occurs with

A glandular fever
B coeliac disease
C cytomegalovirus infections with mononucleosis
D in lymphatic leukaemia
E in coeliac disease

## 2.3 Gynaecomastia may occur with

A spironolactone administration
B malnutrition
C digitalis therapy
D metoclopramide treatment
E cimetidine therapy

## 2.4 In a patient with active tuberculosis of the lungs

A isoniazid could cause a peripheral neuropathy
B treatment with rifampicin may cause disturbance of liver function tests
C streptomycin treatment must always be supplemented by pyridoxine to prevent pyridoxine deficiency
D if ethambutol is prescribed, the patient must be seen by an ophthalmologist
E corticosteroids should be prescribed during the initial phase of antituberculous treatment

2.1   A **False**   rifampicin, isoniazid and pyrazinamide are the
                     bacteriocidal drugs of choice in the UK
      B **False**   para-aminosalicylic acid (PAS) is now obsolete in this
                     country; it is toxic: see for yourself in the books
      C **True**    this is so even if a strain is resistant to isoniazid in
                     vitro
      D **True**    this was common in milliary tuberculosis
      E **True**

2.2   A **True**    high frequency of macular and maculopapular rashes
      B **False**
      C **True**    just like Epstein-Barr virus mononucleosis
                     (glandular fever)
      D **True**    not as widely appreciated as A and C above
      E **False**

2.3   A **True**    due to antiandrogenic activity
      B **False**   however, in malnutrition breasts are preserved until
                     very late, e.g. anorexia nervosa
      C **True**    with digoxin, can be circumvented by giving
                     digitoxin which has no antiandrogen action
      D **False**
      E **True**    uncertain mechanism but cimetidine binds to
                     androgen receptors

2.4   A **True**    isoniazid combines chemically with pyridoxine so
                     causing pyridoxine-deficiency neuropathy (less
                     common in fast acetylators of isoniazid)
      B **True**    common. This may not reflect hepatotoxicity.
                     Rifampicin is an enzyme-inducer and so may
                     increase alkaline phosphatase and gamma-glutamyl
                     transpeptidase because of this property
      C **False**   pyridoxine is given to prevent deficiency with
                     isoniazid
      D **True**    ethambutol causes a retinopathy
      E **False**   corticosteroid treatment may reactivate latent
                     pulmonary tuberculosis

**2.5    Early diagnosis may lead to effective treatment in which of the following diseases?**

A    osteoporosis
B    hypertension
C    carcinoma of the colon
D    motor neurone disease
E    ocular cataracts

**2.6    In a patient with tuberculous meningitis**

A    the cerebrospinal fluid glucose may be low
B    computerised axial tomography may produce abnormal scans
C    intrathecal ampicillin should be given
D    inappropriate secretion of antidiuretic hormone may occur
E    logical treatment would be rifampicin combined with isoniazid and pyrazinamide

**2.7    In the elderly**

A    L-Dopa may cause an acute confusional state independent of the underlying Parkinsons disease
B    a small dose of beta-blocker is the drug treatment of choice in hypertension
C    benzodiazepines are relatively contraindicated
D    a mild to moderate increase in serum alkaline phosphatase suggests excessive alcohol consumption
E    normal adult doses of nebulized beta-agonists are used in the treatment of asthma

**2.8    A male patient with pulmonary tuberculosis is admitted to hospital. During the course of antituberculous treatment of this patient**

A    rifampicin may colour the urine red
B    if he is a fast acetylator of isoniazid, he has an increased risk of isoniazid-induced hepatitis
C    rifampicin may cause deafness
D    a severe skin reaction at the site of a Mantoux test warrants systemic corticosteroids
E    a history of alcoholism suggests that compliance may be a problem

2.5  A **False**   treatment has little effect on the disease at any stage except for oestrogen replacement postmenopause

B **True**   early treatment significantly reduces the secondary damage to organs and prevents strokes, retinopathy, renal and heart failure

C **True**   early surgical excision improves 5-year survival and may be curative

D **False**   there is no treatment

E **False**   cataract surgery is not indicated until the cataract has 'matured' and interferes with vision

2.6  A **True**   also c.s.f. protein is raised and a lymphocytosis may occur

B **True**   hydrocephalus, oedema, exudate over the gyri, basal enhancement and periventricular lucencies

C **False**

D **True**

E **True**   pyrazinamide is especially useful (instead of ethambutol) because, like rifampicin and isoniazid, it is bacteriocidal and crosses the blood-brain barrier

2.7  A **True**   this adverse reaction may occur as the dose is increased; in confusion in the elderly one should always exclude other common causes such as infection and heart failure

B **False**   a small dose of thiazide diuretic is still probably more effective; beta-blockers are as diabetogenic as thiazides and may cause heart failure

C **True**   elderly patients are more sensitive to benzodiazepines and other centrally-active drugs compared with younger adults and may become confused

D **False**   it suggests Paget's disease of the bone

E **True**

2.8  A **True**   patients should always be warned of this

B **True**   fast and slow-acetylators respectively have greater risk of chronic hepatitis or peripheral neuropathy during isoniazid treatment

C **False**   streptomycin, an aminoglycoside, is the antituberculous drug which is oxotoxic

D **False**   a severe local reaction needs only topical steroid; systemic steroids may worsen the tuberculosis

E **True**   poor compliance is an important cause of treatment failure; social factors are important in tuberculosis and its treatment

**2.9   The following drug/situation combinations are to be avoided**
  A   chlorpropamide and renal impairment
  B   propranolol and breast feeding
  C   paracetamol and the first trimester of pregnancy
  D   indomethacin and hypertension
  E   amitriptyline and diets high in cheese

**2.10   Long-term frusemide treatment can**
  A   cause metabolic alkalosis
  B   produce a macrocytic anaemia in some patients
  C   make epileptics on phenytoin worse because of
     displacement of protein-binding of phenytoin
  D   increase blood glucose in some individuals
  E   synergise with cephaloridine or gentamicin in treatment of
     severe infections, e.g. severe pyelonephritis

**2.11   Photosensitivity may occur in**
  A   treatment of sinusitis with doxycycline (vibramycin)
  B   moduretic (combined amiloride and hydrochlorthiazide) in
     essential hypertension
  C   treatment of psoriasis with methotrexate
  D   treatment of epilepsy with primidone
  E   treatment of schizophrenia with depot chlorpromazine

2.9  A **True**     unlike most sulphonylureas chlorpropamide is
                    excreted mostly unchanged in the urine; there is risk
                    of serious hypoglycaemia in chronic renal failure

     B **False**    the amount of propranolol available to the infant via
                    the breast-milk is too small to be harmful

     C **False**    paracetamol seems safe. Aspirin, however, has been
                    implicated as a cause of congenital malformations,
                    perhaps linked to its ability to acetylate proteins, cf.
                    thalidomide which also acylates proteins

     D **True**     non-steroidal anti-inflammatory drugs which are
                    cyclo-oxygenase inhibitors decrease the effects of
                    diuretics and beta-antagonists. Indomethacin raises
                    blood pressure in normal and antihypertensive
                    subjects, presumably by blocking synthesis of
                    vasodilatory postaglandins and causing salt and
                    water retention

     E **False**    monoamine oxidase inhibitors, not tricyclic
                    antidepressants like amitriptyline, block the intestinal
                    oxidation of indirectly-acting sympathomimetic
                    amines like tyramine so producing the 'cheese'
                    reaction — hypertension caused by catecholamine
                    release

2.10 A **True**     sodium and potassium depletion can also occur

     B **False**    one diurotic, triamterene, can because it is a folate-
                    antagonist

     C **False**

     D **True**

     E **False**    dangerous side-effect in impaired renal function is
                    renal failure caused by simultaneous use of
                    cephaloridine or gentamicin and a loop-diuretic

2.11 A **True**     tetracyclines (lipid-soluble) enter skin and are
                    conjugated ring systems which absorb u.v. light

     B **True**     thiazide diuretics may cause photosensitive rashes

     C **False**    but photosensitivity may occur in psoriatic patients
                    taking methoxypsoralen (meladinine) in combination
                    with PUVA treatment

     D **False**

     E **True**     phenothiazines as a group can cause photosensitivity

**2.12  Hirsuitism is a recognised side-effect of**

A   long-term coumarin treatment
B   prolonged use of intravenous heparin
C   treatment of schizophrenia with long-term phenothiazines
D   a combination of flurbiprofen and D-penicillamine in rheumatoid arthritis
E   combined treatment of hypertension with timolol and minoxidil

**2.13  Potassium supplements may be needed in combination with the following drugs**

A   spironolactone
B   the diuretic triamterene
C   carbenoxolone
D   acetazolamide
E   amiloride

**2.14  The combined oral contraceptive pill may cause**

A   hirsuitism
B   hypertension
C   alopecia
D   photosensitivity
E   acne vulgaris

**2.15  The following drugs may cause a drug-induced connective tissue disease**

A   sulphasalazine
B   isoniazid
C   ibuprofen
D   hydralazine
E   phenytoin

**2.16  Griseofulvin**

A   is fungicidal rather than fungistatic
B   if used to treat nail fungal infections usually cures the condition within 7–10 days of starting treatment
C   is active against anaerobic bacteria
D   can cause facial flushing if alcohol is taken by a patient treated with griseofulvin
E   acts by interfering with microbial nucleic acid metabolism

2.12 A **False**
   B **False**   may cause alopecia
   C **False**
   D **False**
   E **True**   minoxidil is the cause, it causes remarkable hair growth over face, scalp, trunk and limbs; this property has been used for alopecia areata (partial or complete scalp hair loss), where oral or topical minoxidil lotion has given encouraging preliminary results

2.13 A **False**   potentially dangerous combination: spironolactone, an aldosterone antagonist, is potassium conserving
   B **False**   also potentially dangerous: triamterene conserves potassium
   C **True**   carbenoxolone has a mineralocorticoid action (sodium retention potassium loss)
   D **True**   one of three causes of hypokalaemic *acidosis* — the other two? — renal tubular acidosis and implantation of ureters into the colon (obsolete operation)
   E **False**   another potentially dangerous combination: amiloride too, conserves potassium

2.14 A **True**   a progestagen effect — those which are alkyl-substituted testosterone derivatives and therefore androgenic
   B **True**   may take weeks to disappear after stopping the pill
   C **False**
   D **False**
   E **True**   due to androgenic effect of certain progestagens

2.15 A **False**
   B **True**
   C **False**
   D **True**   slow acetylators at greatest risk — the risk is less but still present if total daily dose is below 200 mg
   E **True**

2.16 A **True**
   B **False**   it enters the nails as they grow, so many weeks or months may be needed for a cure
   C **False**   we were trying to confuse you with the antifungal clotrimazole which is active against some bacteria
   D **False**
   E **True**

**2.17  In febrile convulsions of infants**

A  aspirin is a preferred antipyretic to paracetamol
B  phenytoin is an effective prophylactic treatment against these convulsions
C  sodium valproate is an effective prophylactic treatment against these convulsions
D  there is a greater risk of temporal lobe epilepsy in adult life if the convulsions are untreated
E  treatment with rectal diazepam may be given by the parents

**2.18  The following measures are useful in decreasing the risk of stroke**

A  daily doses of soluble aspirin
B  treatment of blood pressure sustained at 140/108 mmHg (lying position) with hydrochlorothiazide
C  addition of warfarin, digitalis in a patient with heart failure in sinus rhythm
D  ACTH injections on alternate days in maturity-onset diabetics (non-insulin-dependent diabetics)
E  sulphinpyrazone treatment

**2.19  In patients with depression**

A  inclusion of placebo treatment in a clinical trial of a new antidepressant drug is a matter of course
B  postural hypotension may be a problem if they are treated with amitriptyline
C  an e.c.g. showing left bundle branch block in a patient contraindicates the use of tricyclic antidepressants
D  blurred vision may occur after treatment with desipramine (desmethylimipramine)
E  measurement of serum lithium concentrations is unnecessary if patients on lithium are seen weekly in outpatients

**2.20  In patients with anxiety neurosis**

A  lofepramine is a good initial treatment
B  treatment with a beta-antagonist will cure the anxiety
C  if a benzodiazepine is chosen for treatment, a clinical response nearly always takes at least 3–4 weeks to detect
D  a nocturnal dose of temazepam is unlikely to produce a hangover effect the following morning
E  diazepam may be given once daily because it has a long elimination half-life

2.17 A **False**   paracetamol is safer because aspirin may be linked
       with Reye's syndrome
    B **False**   phenobarbitone and valproate are used in
       prophylaxis
    C **True**    treatment of choice
    D **True**    due to hippocamal damage
    E **True**    safe and effective

2.18 A **True**   exact dose and frequency are controversial but
       40 mg daily is probably enough — it is convenient to
       use paediatric soluble aspirin 1 tablet (75 mg) daily
    B **True**    prevention of stroke has been proven by treatment of
       diastolic blood pressure of > 105 mmHg
    C **False**   digitalisation and warfarin are only appropriate if the
       patient is in atrial fibrillation
    D **False**   would worsen the diabetes (steroid secretion) and so
       (?) worsen the hyperlipidaemia
    E **True**    an alternative if aspirin cannot be tolerated

2.19 A **False**   a placebo is needed to prove efficacy but raises
       ethical issues because of the risk of suicide
    B **True**
    C **True**    this is little known but tricyclics increase the PR
       interval and block conduction in the bundle of His so
       could convert bundle branch block to complete block
    C **True**    an anticholinergic side-effect
    E **False**   measurement of serum lithium is mandatory

2.20 A **False**   lofepramine is an antidepressant drug
    B **False**   beta-antagonists may make people feel better but do
       so by alleviating peripheral symptoms of anxiety,
       they do not cure the underlying cause
    C **False**   the response may be immediate. It is in depression
       treated with tricyclics that a response may require
       3–4 weeks to develop
    D **True**    temazepam has a short half-life and so does not
       usually cause a hangover the day after
    E **True**    especially in the elderly. In chronic usage a great deal
       is converted to N-desmethyldiazepam an active
       metabolite also with a long half-life (about 55 hours)

# Chapter 3

**3.1 In which of the following circumstances can drugs cause renal damage?**

- A use of benzathine penicillin to treat gonorrhoea
- B use of tetracycline date-stamped 1982
- C intravenous amphotericin B given for fungal endocarditis
- D amoxycillin for urinary tract infection
- E ipratropium bromide combined with salbutamol

**3.2 Diabetic candidal vulvitis can effectively be treated with**

- A topical gentamicin cream
- B amphotericin B cream topically
- C intramuscular griseofulvin
- D high-dose nystatin
- E topical clotrimazole cream

**3.3 Patients may suffer withdrawal effects when they abruptly cease**

- A long-term use of oral codeine phosphate for chronic diarrhoea
- B atenolol taken for two years for hypertension
- C long-term tetracycline for acne vulgaris
- D in rheumatoid when long-term aspirin is replaced with indomethacin;
- E clonidine used to treat hypertension for six months

**3.4 Nitrazepam, a benzodiazepine**

- A should not be given at night in chronic bronchitis
- B is a better, shorter-acting hypnotic than diazepam
- C predisposes to deep venous thrombosis
- D must be prescribed with caution in elderly patients
- E can induce liver microsomal hydroxylase enzymes

3.1  A **False**    penicillins are non-toxic but in allergic patients can cause a glomerulorephritis

B **True**    outdated tetracycline can cause acute tubular necrosis

C **True**    amphotericin is nephrotoxic (focal glomerulonephritis could also occur from the endocarditis)

D **False**    even when given to patients with impaired renal function

E **False**    trick question

3.2  A **False**    gentamicin is antibacterial not antifungal. Allergy is a problem with topical antibiotics

B **True**    this drug is safe when used topically

C **False**    rubbish — no such preparation exists and systemic treatment is not indicated

D **False**    nystatin is not absorbed orally but would be useful to eradicate candida from the anal canal where it often occurs

E **False**    miconazole, a related compound, is also effective

3.3  A **True**    codeine phosphate is an opiate and is well absorbed

B **True**    sudden cessation of beta-antagonists can cause tachycardia, arrhythmias and even angina, although it is not clear if this is a true withdrawal syndrome or merely the recurrence of the angina

C **False**    worsening of the acne on stopping tetracycline is due to the underlying causes

D **False**    indomethacin has a similar antiprostaglandin effect

E **True**    clonidine probably does not result in withdrawal symptoms after a single dose but any repeated dose regimen must be gradually withdrawn to prevent rebound hypertension

3.4  A **True**    sedatives can dangerously depress respiration in those patients who have chronic hypercapnoca

B **False**    it is just as long-lasting

C **False**    no benzodiazepine has been implicated in deep venous thrombosis

D **True**    the elderly may show increased sensitivity to hypnotics, sedatives and anxiolytics

E **False**    Do not confuse benzodiazepines with the enzyme-inducing barbiturates

**3.5 The following chemotherapeutic drugs are effective treatment in the infection indicated**

A high-dose tetracycline for *Plasmodium malariae*
B metronidazole in *Entamoeba histolytica* hepatic abcess
C chloroquine for *Giardia lamblia*
D vancomycin for *Clostridium difficile*
E phenoxymethylpenicillin for penicillinase-producing staphylococci

**3.6 Angina pectoris can effectively be treated with**

A topical glyceryl trinitrate
B sublingual isosorbide dinitrate
C nebulized terbutaline sulphate
D oral nifedipine
E intravenous domperidone

**3.7 Use of a combined oestrogen-progestrogen contraceptive pill is unwise in young females with**

A spasmodic (primary) dysmenorrhoea
B rheumatoid arthritis
C recent treatment for depression
D history of recurrent migraine
E history of Crohn's disease

**3.8 Palpitations may be a side-effect of the following**

A small dose of bendrofluazide for hypertension
B alpha-methyldopa for hypertension
C nifedipine for angina
D oxprenolol in hypertension
E hydralazine for hypertension

3.5  A **False**
    B **True**    dehydroemetine is an alternative but is more nauseating and is cardiotoxic. Diloxanide furoate is given after metronidazole to kill any remaining encysted forms of amoebae
    C **True**    metronidazole is more commonly used for giardia
    D **True**    this antibiotic is not absorbed but acts against *Clostridium difficile*, which is confined to the gut. Metronidazole has also been shown to be effective. *Clostridium difficile* overgrowth occurs in pseudomembranous colitis.
    E **False**    methicillin, cloxacillin or flucloxacillin are correct choices.

3.6  A **True**    as ointment impregnated plasters/silicone discs
    B **True**    both glyceryl trinitrate and isosorbide dinitrate can be given sublingually
    C **False**    beta-agonist vasodilation and tachycardia may worsen the attack
    D **True**    calcium antagonists are new antianginals
    E **False**    domperidone is a new dopamine-antagonist antiemetic

3.7  A **False**    combined pill may be useful treatment
    B **False**
    C **True**    the pill may exacerbate depression
    D **True**    the pill may cause migraine
    E **False**

3.8  A **False**    thiazides act as vasodilators in hypertension, but do not produce palpitations like minoxidil, hydralazine and calcium antagonists
    B **False**
    C **True**    nifedipine is a potent peripheral vasodilator
    D **False**    oxprenolol is a beta-antagonist and a partial beta-agonist but will not cause tachycardia (except in rare autonomic degeneration syndromes like the Shy Drager syndrome)
    E **True**    hydralazine is a potent peripheral vasodilator and may cause palpitations, flushing and headache; simultaneous use of a beta-antagonist can prevent the tachycardia

**3.9    In an asthmatic patient with an acute severe asthmatic attack**

A    intravenous aminophylline is useful
B    100% oxygen is contraindicated since it may depress respiratory drive
C    the treatment of choice is intravenous dexamethasone
D    intravenous atenolol, which is cardioselective, is useful for treating tachycardia
E    an urgent chest X-ray is indicated

**3.10   A non-depolarising blockade of the neuromuscular junction is produced during anaesthesia by**

A    physostigmine
B    succinylcholine (suxamethonium)
C    D-tubocurarine
D    pancuronium
E    atropine

**3.11   Physical drug dependance may occur after prolonged use of the following drugs**

A    ergotamine preparations for migraine
B    codeine phosphate in chronic diarrhoea
C    loperamide treatment of irritable bowel syndrome diarrhoea
D    lomotil (diphenoxylate and atropine) for chronic diarrhoea
E    distalgesic for osteoarthritic pain

**3.12   After an overdosage of diamorphine (heroin, diacetyl morphine)**

A    the pupils will be widely dilated
B    a toxic confusional state may be present
C    severe left ventricular failure is common
D    intravenous naloxone can be life saving
E    an alkaline diuresis enhances drug-clearance

3.9 A **True** as a bolus followed by a continuous infusion
B **False** 100% oxygen is needed; if arterial $Po_2$ does not rise with 100% oxygen, intubation and IPPV may be needed. Only in patients with hypercapnoea is 100% oxygen contraindicated
C **False** Intravenous corticosteroids are needed but they are not the treatment of choice
D **False** tachycardia is a physiological response and does not need treatment; cardioselective beta-antagonists can still worsen bronchoconstriction
E **True** especially to exclude a pneumothorax or infection

3.10 A **False** physostigmine an anticholinesterase reverses competitive neuromuscular blockade by increasing acetylcholine concentrations at the neuromuscular junction
B **False** suxamethonium causes a depolarising blockade
C **True**
D **True** pancuronium is beginning to replace D-tubocurarine for major surgery
E **False** atropine is an anti-muscarinic drug and does not act at nicotinic acetylcholine receptors which occur at the muscular junction and which are blocked by tubocurarine and pancuronium

3.11 A **False**
B **True** codeine is an opiate and is absorbed
C **False** loperamide is an opiate, but is almost entirely unabsorbed and is a safe and potent antidiarrhoeal
D **True** diphenoxylate is an opiate and is absorbed
E **True** distalgesic contains the opiate dextropropoxyphene

3.12 A **False** narcotics cause constricted pupils
B **True**
C **False**
D **True**
E **False** only of use in aspirin and barbiturate renal clearance

**3.13    The following are true general statements about pharmacokinetic properties of drugs**

A    highly plasma protein-bound drugs have a very large volume of distribution
B    lipid-soluble beta-antagonist cause bad dreams more often than water-soluble beta-antagonists
C    gastrointestinal absorption of lipid soluble drugs occurs more readily than water soluble drugs
D    hepatic drug metabolism often involves conversion of a water-soluble into a more lipid-soluble drug
E    renal failure markedly increases the plasma protein-binding of drugs

**3.14    The following drugs are appropriate treatment for the conditions named**

A    mycoplasma ('atypical', 'viral') pneumonia — metronidazole
B    familial mediterranean fever — colchicine
C    streptococcal cellulitis of theleg — benzylpenicillin
D    nephrogenic diabetes insipidus — chlorpropamide
E    tinea cruris — griseofulvin

**3.15    Inhaled drugs may produce the following effects**

A    beclomethasone dipropionate — palpitations and flushing
B    24% oxygen — respiratory depression in chronic bronchitis
C    100% oxygen — respiratory depression in acute asthma
D    salbutamol — fine muscular tremor
E    halothane — a low incidence of postoperative nausea and vomiting

**3.16    Raynaud's phenomenon (decreased blood flow in the extremities) may occur as a side-effect of**

A    oxprenolol
B    ethanol abuse
C    phentolamine
D    ergotamine
E    naftidrofuryl (praxilene) oxalate

**3.17    In a patient treated with isoniazid**

A    peripheral neuropathy may occur
B    the antibacterial action of the drug is antagonised by simultaneous administration of rifampicin
C    exacerbation of epilepsy may be a problem
D    hepatitis is more likely if the patient is a fast acetylator
E    hepatic enzyme induction will result rendering the low dose (25, 30 microgram) oestrogen contraceptive pill ineffective

3.13 A **False**    tight plasma protein binding holds drugs in the vascular compartment so that the volume of distribution is about 4–5 l

   B **True**    lipid-soluble substances more easily cross the blood brain barrier, e.g. pindolol, one of the most lipid soluble beta-antagonists causes bad dreams more often than atenolol

   C **True**    lipid-soluble drugs dissolve in lipid membranes and are less likely to be ionized than water-soluble drugs

   D **False**    production of more water-soluble metabolites is the rule

   E **False**    decreased plasma protein concentrations and less binding make patients more sensitive to some drugs, e.g. diazoxide, phenytoin

3.14 A **False**    tetracycline is needed
   B **True**    colchicine prevents relapses (Honours standard!)
   C **True**
   D **True**    thiazide diuretics are also of use (well done if you got this one)
   E **False**    cotrimazole or miconazole topically is correct, systemic griseofulvon is OK for nail or scalp ringworm

3.15 A **False**    beclomethasone is a corticosteroid
   B **False**    in general 24% or less oxygen is needed
   C **False**    100% oxygen is needed
   D **True**    stimulation of skeletal muscle beta-receptors
   E **True**    a great advantage of halothane

3.16 A **True**    of any beta-agonist including cardioselective ones
   B **False**    ethanol is a vasodilator
   C **False**    alpha-antagonism would not cause vasoconstriction
   D **True**    a danger of overdose in obstetrics and in antimigraine preparations
   E **False**    naftidrofuryl is used as a peripheral vasodilator

3.17 A **True**    greater risk in 'slow acetylators'. Pyridoxine deficiency may enhance this risk so pyridoxine is coprescribed
   B **False**    rifampicin is usually prescribed with isoniazid for tuberculosis
   C **False**
   D **True**
   E **False**    do not confuse with rifampicin, the antitubercle drug, which is an enzyme inducer

**3.18    Renal failure increases the risk of side-effects with the following drugs**

A    phenoxymethylpenicillin
B    frusemide
C    tetracycline
D    digoxin
E    diazoxide

**3.19    The yellow card adverse drug reactions monitoring scheme linked to the Committee of Safety of Medicines**

A    makes it illegal for doctors not to report suspected side-effects
B    allows a precise estimate of all drug reactions occurring in current medical practice in Britain
C    is largely controlled by the Association of the British Pharmaceutical Industry (ABPI)
D    allows doctors to make important notifications of suspected adverse reactions to any drugs
E    has been effective in the past in alerting medical practitioners to certain dangerous effects

**3.20    A patient with a pulmonary embolus is given an anticoagulating dose of warfarin. In this patient**

A    anticoagulation will be effective within about 2–3 hours after warfarin ingestion
B    heparin is contraindicated because of the risk of bleeding
C    prophylactic cimetidine should be given to decrease risk of haematemesis
D    hepatic synthesis of coagulation factors II, VII, IX and X will be decreased
E    if allergy to warfarin occurs, phenindione is a useful alternative

3.18 A **False**    penicillins are cleared in the urine but their therapeutic index is so high that retention in the body is not usually a problem

B **True**    risk of ototoxicity (vestibular and auditory)

C **False**    tetracycline is also concentrated and excreted in the bile

D **True**    blood concentrations need careful checking

E **True**    decreased protein binding increases its effectiveness (one author has seen three patients with renal failure blinded after rapid i.v. boluses of diazoxide to treat hypertension — occipital cortex infarction)

3.19 A **False**    reporting is entirely voluntary — please do so nonetheless

B **False**    many reactions go unnoticed, or worse — unreported

C **False**    though the ABPI might wish it so

D **True**

E **True**    practolol oculomucocutaneous syndrome is one example

3.20 A **False**    takes 36–48 hours for stores of II, VII, IX, X to decrease

B **False**    heparin is needed for immediate anticoagulation (heparin's antiplatelet aggregating effect is of help here)

C **False**    avoid cimetidine since it decreases liver enzyme inactivation of warfarin

D **True**

E **True**    phenindione is a member of the indanedione group of anticoagulants, its action is similar to warfarin

# Chapter 4

**4.1** **Amiodarone**

**A** decreases heart rate by increasing conduction in the bundle velocity in the bundle of His

**B** is effective only in ventricular arrhythmias

**C** is contraindicated in Wolff-Parkinson-White syndrome because it causes increased automaticity of the myocardium

**D** may cause lens opacities

**E** must be given twice daily because its half-life is short

**4.2** **The following are useful ways of monitoring the effect of the given drugs on the specific disease processes mentioned in each case**

**A** blood glycosylated haemoglobin for diabetes treated with glibenclamide

**B** blood c-peptide concentrations for diabetes mellitus treated with chlorpropamide

**C** blood fructosamine bound to albumin for diabetes mellitus treated with insulin

**D** blood pressure (sitting and standing) for angina pectoris treated with propranolol

**E** fit chart for idiopathic epilepsy treated with phenytoin

**4.3** **A 67 year old female takes tenoretic (atenolol 100 mg plus chlorthalidone 25 mg) one tablet daily for hypertension, glibenclamide 2.5 mg once daily (manufacturer's recommended doses 2.5 to 15 mg per day), metformin 500 mg three times a day (maximum dose recommended 850 mg in 12 hours). Her blood glucose before and after breakfast (0800 h) and dinner (1900 h) are 7 and 8, 6 and 9 mmoles per litre respectively. The following are true of this patient**

**A** the tenoretic might have contributed to her diabetes

**B** the metformin should be stopped

**C** the glibenclamide dose should be increased

**D** the metformin dose should be increased

**E** it would be reasonable to stop all the drugs and check the blood sugar profile

4.1  A **False**   heart rate falls mainly as a result of direct action on
                   the SA node
     B **False**   effective against atrial and ventricular arrhythmias
     C **False**   it is effective treatment; verapamil may also be used
     D **True**    microdeposits in the lower third of the cornea may
                   develop during therapy, but disappear after stopping
                   the drug
     E **False**   the half-life is several weeks

4.2  A **True**   glycosylated haemoglobin reflects long term
                   (minimum 6 weeks) blood glucose control
     B **False**   C-peptide does reflect the amount of active insulin
                   secreted but its measurement is a research tool
                   rather than a yardstick for judging clinical response
     C **True**    albumin becomes glycosylated just like haemoglobin
                   and albumin bound fructosamine has recently been
                   shown useful to assess glucose control of periods
                   from 24 hours to 1 month
     D **False**   obviously the frequency of anginal pain and possibly
                   the amount of glyceryl trinitrate consumed is a
                   measure of the effect of propranolol on the angina
     E **True**    out-patients or their relatives can keep a diary; useful
                   for research too

4.3  A **True**   thiazides are diabetogenic
     B **True**   the dose of glibenclamide is small so adding a
                   diguanide to the treatment is illogical
     C **False**
     D **False**
     E **True**   one should stop tenoretic gradually (change to
                   conventional atenolol and reduce the dose) the
                   others can be stopped immediately. It may be that
                   without the thiazide in the tenoretic there will be no
                   diabetes or that control will be adequate on diet
                   alone

**4.4    Sulphinpyrazone**

A    inhibits platelet aggregation
B    is a powerful vasodilating agent so improving cerebral blood flow and preventing strokes
C    is contraindicated if colchicine is administered
D    inhibits xanthine oxidase
E    when given to patients blood counts should be monitored

**4.5    The following drugs are recognized causes of constipation**

A    propranolol
B    dextropropoxyphene
C    nefopam
D    vernpamil
E    L-thyroxine

**4.6    A patient finds difficulty in co-ordinating breathing sufficiently with actuation of a pressurised aerosol inhaler delivering a beta-agonist bronchodilator. The following are appropriate steps to take in rectifying the situation**

A    immediate change to an oral form of the bronchodilator instead of the inhaler.
B    use of a breath-activated inhaler
C    use of a spacer device with the inhaler
D    education of the patient in inhaler technique
E    use of a nebuliser inhaling device to produce an aqueous aerosol of the bronchodilator

**4.7    The following are true of beta-adrenoceptor blocking drugs in general**

A    they may cause a tachycardia in large doses
B    given in the first to the third years after a heart attack they decrease mortality
C    long term treatment with these drugs prevents or decreases the extent of coronary heart disease
D    inhaled formulations of the drugs are available to produce bronchodilation in asthma
E    combination with a vasodilator/calcium channel antagonist may cause postural hypotension

**4.8    The following drugs given alone are useful for treatment of hypertension**

A    amiloride
B    propanolol
C    captopril
D    triamterene
E    ketanserin

4.4 A **True**   the clinical significance of this is unclear
    B **False**   it is not a vasodilator and does not prevent strokes
    C **False**   there is no interaction between sulphinpyrazone and colchicine, but uricosuric drugs are usually avoided during the acute phase of gout
    D **False**   allopurinol is the only xanthine oxidase inhibitor used clinically
    E **True**   blood dyscrasias may occur after short or long treatment

4.5 A **False**   beta-antagonists may cause diarrhoea
    B **True**   often occurs with combination analgesics (eg. distalgesic, co-proxamol) especially in the elderly
    C **False**   freedom from this side-effect is a good property of this useful analgesic
    D **True**   not as well known as its cardiac side-effects
    E **False**   in large doses may cause diarrhoea

4.6 A **False**   oral formulations of currently-available bronchodilators tend to give more peripheral side-effects and less bronchodilatation than inhaled types
    B **True**   two currently available are for terbutaline ('Bricanyl turbohaler') and salbutamol ('Aerolin inhaler') both are rather expensive
    C **True**   cheap and effective either as a plastic pull-out device on the inhaler or as a 'volumatic' flask
    D **True**
    E **True**   but care needs to be taken because the dose delivered is large relative to an inhaled puff

4.7 A **False**   they cause bradycardia
    B **True**   shown for a number of drugs including timolol, atenolol
    C **False**   there is no evidence for this, the reverse might be true for they reduce the level of High Density Lipoproteins in blood
    D **False**
    E **True**   reports have been published for combinations with nifedipine to treat hypertension

4.8 A **False**   this acts on the distal tubule lumen to block sodium-potassium exchange and so is useful for conserving potassium but is a very weak antihypertensive
    B **True**
    C **True**
    D **False**   similar to A above, is useful only in combination with thiazides to conserve potassium
    E **True**   This 5-HT receptor antagonist lowers blood pressure

**4.9    Synthetic oestrogen derivatives**
A    may cause deep venous thrombosis
B    may result in arterial thrombosis in the nervous system
C    may induce remission in postmenopausal breast carcinoma
D    are drugs of choice to suppress lactation in the puerperium
E    are metabolized more rapidly when isoniazid is prescribed simultaneously

**4.10   The following drugs are associated with the side-effects listed**
A    amantadine and livedo reticularis
B    barbiturates and blistering skin lesions
C    corticosteroids and skin rashes
D    ampicillin and fixed drug eruption
E    nitrofurantoin and peripheral neuropathy

**4.11   Metronidazole is a useful drug in the treatment of infections due to**
A    *Giardia lamblia*
B    *Eschericia coli* gastroenteritis
C    *Plasmodium malariae*
D    *Entamoeba histolytica*
E    non-specific urethritis

**4.12   In a patient with asthma**
A    nasal polyps suggest that aspirin may be contraindicated
B    ipratropium bromide synergises with the action of beta-adrenoceptor agonists
C    acute attacks may require intravenous propranolol if there is a tachycardia
D    oxygen is not needed
E    if the $P_a co_2$ rises, then intermittent positive pressure ventilation may be needed

**4.13   Isoniazid**
A    is an hepatic enzyme inducer
B    may be associated with peripheral neuropathy
C    may be associated with chronic hepatitis
D    can cause convulsions
E    demonstrates bimodal distribution of drug metabolism

4.9    A **True**      usually when other risk factors present, e.g. smoking
       B **True**      also an increased risk of myocardial infarction
       C **True**      in contrast to premenopausal types which may be
                       oestrogen dependent
       D **False**     bromocriptine is now the drug of choice
       E **False**     enzyme inducers such as rifampicin increase the
                       metabolism

4.10   A **True**      a curious erythematous mottling rash
       B **True**      characteristic barbiturate blisters seen in overdose
       C **False**
       D **False**
       E **True**

4.11   A **True**      this organism infects the upper small bowel
       B **False**     antibiotic not indicated
       C **False**     antimalarial drugs indicated
       D **True**      active against all forms of the organism
       E **False**     the only sexually-transmitted organism against
                       which it is active is *Trichomonas vaginalis*

4.12   A **True**
       B **False**     the combined effect is not greater than the sum of
                       the individual effects
       C **False**     propranolol and all beta-antagonists are
                       contraindicated in all cases of asthma
       D **False**     100% oxygen is needed
       E **True**      increased $P_a$ co$_2$ suggests that ventilatory drive is
                       decreasing

4.13   A **False**     it is an enzyme inhibitor, important in patients on
                       treatment for epilepsy
       B **True**      isoniazid forms hydrazones with pyridoxine and so
                       may cause pyridoxine deficiency, which may be the
                       cause of the neuropathy
       C **True**      associated with fast acetylators of the drug
       D **True**      this is usually seen in patients with a history of
                       convulsions
       E **True**

## 4.14 The following drugs may be given in pregnancy

A    ampicillin for lower urinary tract infections
B    tetracycline for urinary tract infections
C    carbimazole for hyperthyroidism
D    methyldopa for pre-eclamptic hypertension
E    warfarin for a deep venous thrombosis

## 4.15 Griseofulvin

A    may cause facial flushing if alcohol is taken
B    increases the action of dicoumarol anticoagulants
C    must not be taken with food since this will slow griseofulvin absorption
D    cures tinea pedis within two weeks of starting treatment
E    is a powerful drug for treatment of chronic candidiasis of the nails

## 4.16 Patients taking a daily dose of predrisolone 60 mg

A    may as a result develop purpura due to thrombocytopenia
B    any of these patients who develop a raised neutrophil polymorph count should be given antibiotics immediately
C    some of these patients may suffer an acute psychosis as a result of the prednisolone
D    these patients may develop hypokalaemia due to the prednisolone
E    some of these patients may develop a weakness of proximal muscle groups

## 4.17 Diarrhoea may occur with

A    dextropropoxyphene and paracetamol combinations
B    treatment of hypertension with guanethidine
C    amitriptyline given long term
D    colchicine treatment of acute gout
E    lithium therapy for severe depression

4.14 A **True**    broad-spectrum antibiotic of choice
     B **False**    harms fetal teeth. Risk of maternal hepatic and renal damage
     C **True**    antithyroid drugs cross the placenta and enter breast milk, may cause fetal and postnatal hypothyroidism — low doses given
     D **True**    beta-antagonists, hydralazine and nifedipine have been used but alpha-methyldopa has had the greatest use and so is probably the safest
     E **False**    warfarin is contraindicated because it causes fetal malformations

4.15 A **False**    there is no antabuse effect, but alcohol should be avoided
     B **False**    reduces the anticoagulant activity, possibly via enzyme induction.
     C **False**    dietary fat increases the absorption of griseofulvin
     D **False**    active only against *Microsporum*, *Trichophyton* and *Epidermophyton* species
     E **False**

4.16 A **False**    purpura may occur with steroids, but steroids do not cause thrombocytopenia
     B **False**    infection should be sought but a polymorph neutrophil leucocytosis can be caused by steroids alone
     C **True**    also seen in patients with Cushing's disease
     D **False**    hypokalaemia may occur due to the mineralocorticoid effect'
     E **True**    corticosteroids cause a proximal myopathy

4.17 A **False**    dextropropoxyphene, like other opiates, tends to cause constipation
     B **True**    a complication of adrenergic neurone blockade
     C **False**    anticholinergic drugs tend to cause constipation
     D **True**    diarrhoea and nausea limit the dose of colchicine which can be given
     E **True**    nausea, vomiting and cramps are other gut symptoms of toxicity

**4.18   Diazepam**

    **A**  when metabolized gives rise only to inactive metabolites

    **B**  is useful to treat effects of increased muscle tone in demyelinating diseases

    **C**  must be given four-hourly for anxiety since it has a half-life of only about two hours

    **D**  is contraindicated in combination with monoamine oxidase inhibitors

    **E**  is a useful drug to treat febrile convulsions in children

**4.19   In a patient with a duodenal ulcer**

    **A**  sucralfate (sucrose octa sulphate) may heal the ulcer

    **B**  ranitidine is superior to cimetidine for treatment

    **C**  ibuprofen treatment of arthritis would be contraindicated

    **D**  cigarettes may have been important in the causation

    **E**  oral ethanol would heal the ulcer

**4.20   In staphylococcal infections**

    **A**  oral benzylpenicillin is preferred to oral cloxacillin because absorption is better with benzylpenicillin

    **B**  flucloxacillin is preferred to cloxacillin when oral therapy is indicated

    **C**  combination therapy including fusidic acid is indicated in osteomyelitis

    **D**  oral methicillin is an alternative to oral cloxacillin

    **E**  clindamycin is active against staphylococci

4.18 A **False**   once-daily dosing is adequate in view of the long
                   half-life of diazepam and its active N-desmethyl
                   metabolite
     B **True**    an alternative antispastic drug would be baclofen or
                   clonazepam
     C **False**   a major metabolite, N-desmethyldiazepam, is active
                   and makes a major contribution to the action of
                   repeated doses of diazepam
     D **False**   monoamine oxidase is not involved in diazepam
                   metabolism
     E **True**    may be given intravenously or rectally to prevent or
                   treat convulsions

4.19 A **True**    good rate of healing similar to $H_2$ antagonists
     B **False**   both drugs heal ulcers
     C **True**    since bleeding from the ulcer may occur
     D **True**
     E **False**   the converse is true!

4.20 A **False**   cloxacillin may be used, although it is poorly
                   absorbed orally; benzylpenicillin is destroyed by
                   gastric acid and must be given parenterally
     B **True**    the bioavailability of flucloxacillin is greater than that
                   of cloxacillin because flucloxacillin is better absorbed
     C **Truc**    fusidic acid has good bone penetration
     D **False**   although similar spectrum of activity to cloxacillin,
                   can only be given intramuscularly, painfully!
     E **True**    it is rarely used for staphylocci now because of the
                   risk of pseudomembraneous colitis; clindamycin is
                   used for anaerobic infections

# Chapter 5

**5.1  In man, the administration of histamine may produce the following effects**

- A  bronchoconstriction
- B  negative chronotropic action
- C  increased secretion of gastric acid
- D  vasodilation
- E  inhibition of intrinsic factor secretion

**5.2  The following are true of antihistamine $H_1$-antagonists**

- A  help relieve itching of skin eruptions in drug allergies
- B  worsen the nausea of Ménière's disease
- C  terfenadine, a new antihistamine, causes very little drowsiness
- D  prochlorperazine can be safely used to treat nausea in pregnancy
- E  cyclizine is preferred to phenothiazine antihistamines to prevent nausea in patients with myocardial infarction

**5.3  Histamine $H_2$-antagonist drugs cause**

- A  decreased oxyntic (parietal) cell secretion
- B  increased rate of gastric emptying because they stimulate gastric antral motility and relax the pylorus
- C  gynaecomastia after prolonged use
- D  the action of warfarin may be potentiated
- E  a common side effect is nausea and vomiting due to medullary chemoreceptor trigger zone stimulation

**5.4  Vomiting may be a troublesome side-effect after use of the following drugs**

- A  propranolol treatment of angina pectoris
- B  use of high-dose parenteral metoclopramide
- C  cisplatin
- D  desferrioxamine
- E  halothane

5.1  A **True**    via $H_1$ receptors
     B **False**   action is positive by direct effect on heart receptors
                   and by baroreceptor reflex due to vasodilatation
     C **True**    via $H_2$ receptors, also increases pepsinogen and
                   intrinsic factor secretion
     D **True**    remember the 'triple response': wheal, flare, oedema
     E **False**   $H_2$-antagonists rather than histamine decrease
                   intrinsic factor secretion

5.2  A **True**    one of their best uses is relief of pruritis
     B **False**   rubbish, they are used to treat Ménière's Disease and
                   motion sickness
     C **True**    you *are* up to date if you got this
     D **False**   nausea of pregancy is a problem; no antinauseant
                   can be given safely in pregnancy
     E **True**    phenothiazine antiemetics increase infarct size in
                   animal models of acute myocardial infarction.
                   Cyclizine prevents nausea induced by opiates given
                   to relieve infarct pain

5.3  A **True**    acid, directly and pepsinogen/intrinsic factor as
                   secondary effects
     B **False**   meant to confuse you with metoclopramide which
                   does have these effects
     C **True**    with cimetidine but not ranitidine
     D **True**    cimetidine (*not* ranitidine) inhibits liver oxidation of
                   warfarin and other drugs
     E **False**

5.4  A **False**   beta-blockers rarely cause gastrointestinal side
                   effects
     B **False**   this regimen is used to prevent nausea associated
                   with cytotoxic drugs
     C **True**    cisplatin, a platinum salt, is infamous in this respect
                   (high-dose metoclopramide inhibits cisplatin-induced
                   nausea)
     D **False**   this chelating agent used in the treatment of iron
                   overload rarely causes gastrointestinal side effects
     E **True**    all anaesthetics can cause nausea/vomiting in the
                   recovery period; halothane has less tendency to do
                   so than others

**5.5    The following are statements about dopamine antagonist drugs such as metoclopramide; which are true?**

A    they are effective in preventing the lactation seen in hyperprolactinaemic states

B    tardive dyskinesia is an occasional side-effect

C    they antagonise the effect of apomorphine on the medullary chemoreceptor trigger-zone

D    may cause nausea and oesophogeal reflux by delaying gastric emptying

E    represent a new approach to treatment of Parkinsonism

**5.6    Antacids are widely used for the treatment of peptic ulcer. The following is true of their use**

A    sodium bicarbonate is a non-systemic antacid

B    aluminium hydroxide can cause troublesome diarrhoea

C    magnesium hydroxide ingestion may produce diarrhoea

D    very high-dose antacid treatment may heal duodenal ulcers

E    high-dose antacid therapy blocks the action of histamine $H_2$-antagonists in healing gastric ulcers

**5.7    A 76-year-old lady presents with a large (3 × 4 cm) raised ulcerating lesion on the flexor surface of her right root; the right inguinal nodes are not palpable. A clinical diagnosis of epithelioma is made. Other signs present are chronic bronchitis and slow atrial fibrillation with warm extremities. Her medication is frusemide, thyroxine and amiloride**

A    the treatment of choice for the epithelioma is topical 5-fluorouracil cream

B    the epithelioma should be excised surgically

C    immediate digitalization is needed

D    a course of treatment with cisplatin (a cytotoxic) is a good alternative to surgery for this lady

E    serum thyroxine values in this lady could indicate thyrotoxicosis

**5.8    A 42-year-old man with rheumatic mitral stenosis is observed to be in atrial fibrillation; there are no signs of cardiac failure**

A    intravenous lignocaine is indicated to slow this man's ventricular rate

B    direct current cardioversion may stop the arrhythmia

C    anticoagulation is contraindicated in this patient because of the risk of bleeding from enlarged pulmonary capillaries

D    prescription of oral frusemide is a sensible precaution against heart failure

E    oral ouabain is preferred to digoxin because it acts more quickly

5.5    A **False**    dopamine agonists will reduce prolactin not
                      dopamine antagonists
       B **True**     especially in children and young adults given
                      metoclopramide
       C **True**     apomorphine produces vomiting and dopamine
                      antagonists are antiemetics by acting on the
                      medullary centre
       D **False**    they increase lower oesophageal sphincter tone and
                      hasten gastric emptying
       E **False**

5.6    A **False**    Na and $HCO_3$ are absorbed and may precipitate heart
                      failure
       B **False**    aluminium is constipating
       C **True**     insoluble magnesium salts formed in small intestine
                      exert an osmotic effect causing diarrhoea (remember
                      magnesium sulphate — Epsom salts — a Victorian
                      purgative!)
       D **True**     shown clearly in clinical trials, but frequency of
                      dosing and quantity needed may make the more
                      expensive $H_2$-antagonists preferable
       E **False**    however, antacids may reduce absorption of
                      cimetidine

5.7    A **False**    5-flurouracil cream can be tried for small cutaneous
                      carcinomata but this epithelioma is too large
       B **True**
       C **False**    atrial fibrillation is slow and no signs of cardiac
                      failure were present. Digoxin is not indicated at all
       D **False**    cisplatin has been successful for testicular tumours
                      but is toxic (especially nauseating), with the
                      decreased renal function of old age
       E **True**     atrial fibrillation and warm extremities could indicate
                      overdosing with thyroxine. Thyroxine and free
                      thyroxine index should be checked regularly anyway

5.8    A **False**    lignocaine is used for ventricular ectopic arrhythmias
       B **True**     atrial fibrillation may be reverted to sinus rhythm.
                      Spontaneous reversion back to atrial fibrillation is
                      common
       C **False**    oral anticoagulants always carry a risk of bleeding
                      and haemoptysis occurs in mitral stenosis, but the
                      anticoagulants probably decrease the risk of
                      thromboembolism
       D **False**    heart failure should be treated as and when it
                      develops
       E **False**    intravenously, digitalisation is faster with ouabain
                      but is seldom used; ouabain is poorly absorbed
                      orally

**5.9    In a 41-year-old male patient with an uncomplicated chronic duodenal ulcer**

A    high oral doses of magnesium hydroxide may heal the ulcer

B    treatment with tripotassium dicitratobismuthate (De nol) would relieve ulcer pain but would be unlikely to heal the ulcer

C    he should be given carbenoxolone as the treatment of choice for healing his ulcer

D    ibuprofen could be given safely to relieve the pain of a sprained ankle

E    he could be given oral cimetidine and must be told to stop cigarette smoking

**5.10    In a patient with severe haematemesis from oesophageal varices with a blood pressure of 60/40 mmHg, the following steps may be taken**

A    immediate transfusion with dextran plasma expander followed by blood sampling for determination of blood group and cross-match

B    he should be given intramuscular cimetidine

C    intravenous ergotamine would decrease the bleeding

D    intravenous vasopressin may be useful

E    a Sengstaken-Blakemore tube can be used to help control bleeding

**5.11    You are called to see, as an emergency, a 6-year-old child who has hot, dry, flushed skin, dry mouth, widely dilated pupils, fever, confusion and tachycardia. The following are likely to be true**

A    he has salicylate poisoning

B    he may have atropine poisoning

C    these symptoms could have occured if he had taken a bottle of antimotion sickness tablets containing cyclizine

D    intravenous physostigmine may reverse the symptoms

E    intravenous naloxone is indicated by the clinical picture

**5.12    In a female patient with acne vulgaris**

A    a course of tetracycline may be of benefit

B    topical dithranol reduces the size of the lesions

C    a change from a combined to a synthetic progestogen-only contraceptive pill would be indicated

D    topical cis-retinoic acid could be indicated

E    salicylsulphonic acid cream (topical) is of use

5.9  A **True**   there is no information, however, about gastric ulcers
     B **False**  this drug heals both gastric and duodenal ulcers and
                  will relieve ulcer pain
     C **False**  carbenoxolone is sometimes used for gastric ulcers
                  (though it heals both types) but has many side-
                  effects
     D **False**  non-steroidal anti-inflammatory drugs may
                  precipitate severe bleeding from the ulcer.
                  Paracetamol could be the first choice
     E **True**   $H_2$-antagonists heal duodenal ulcers, smoking
                  worsens them (and inhibits the effect of cimetidine).
                  Stopping smoking alone may heal ulcers

5.10 A **False**  blood sample first since dextrans interfere with
                  cross-match. Haemacell is a plasma expander that
                  does not affect crossmatching
     B **False**  intravenous $H_2$-antagonists have been given, but
                  their use is still controversial
     C **False**  ergotamine is used to control postpartum uterine
                  bleeding
     D **True**   constricting the splanchnic vascular bed may
                  decrease blood loss
     E **True**   by direct pressure from the oesophageal lumen

5.11 A **False**  sweating, hyperventilation and tinnutis would be
                  expected in salicylate overdose
     B **True**   these features are typical anticholinergic effects
     C **True**   cyclizine like many $H_1$-antihistamines is an
                  anticholinergic so it is used in motion sickness;
                  sedation may also occur
     D **True**   if anticholinergic poisoning was the cause
     E **False**  naloxone is a narcotic antagonist. Constricted pupils
                  bradycardia and hypothemia occur in opiate
                  poisoning

5.12 A **True**   several antibiotics have been shown to be beneficial.
                  Erythromycin and tetracycline are commonly used;
                  cotrimoxazole works too
     B **False**  dithranol is used for psoriasis
     C **False**  most progestagens are 17-alpha alkyl nortestosterore
                  derivatives and cause acne
     D **True**   useful in severe resistant cases. Reduces sebum
                  production
     E **True**   an old-fashioned keratolytic agent that still works!

**5.13  A patient with acute exacerbation of chronic bronchitis was treated with nebulised salbutamol; he noticed a fine tremor of his hands and his blood pressure was 180/60 mmHg**

 A   the tremor could be due to salbutamol
 B   the tremor could be due to hypercapnoea
 C   treatment with a pressurised inhaler would decrease the chance of side-effects from salbutamol
 D   the high systolic pressure should be treated with propranolol
 E   phentolamine should be at hand in case of salbutamol overdose

**5.14  In obstetric practice the use of the following drugs is well accepted**

 A   salbutamol for induction of labour
 B   ergotamine for postpartum haemorrhage
 C   ergotamine for delay in second stage labour
 D   bromocriptine to suppress lactation
 E   alpha-methyldopa for pre-eclamptic raised blood pressure

**5.15  Tachycardia may be a side-effect of treatment with the following drugs**

 A   nifedipine
 B   atenolol
 C   spironolactone
 D   bendrofluazide
 E   minoxidil

**5.16  Myopathy may be a side-effect of**

 A   spironolactone
 B   bumetanide
 C   loperamide
 D   labetalol
 E   triamcinolone

**5.17  Clonazepam (7-chloro-nitrazepam)**

 A   is useful in the treatment of status asthmatics
 B   worsens grand mal epilepsy
 C    effectively suppresses myoclonic jerks (myoclonus)
 D   prevents the antihypotensive action of debrisoquine
 E   may cause sedation

5.13 A **True**   stimulation of skeletal muscle beta$_2$-receptors
 B **False**   $CO_2$ retention causes a tremor similar to the tremor
of liver disease, a coarse flapping tremor, not a fine
tremor
 C **True**   the dose would be considerably greater via a
nebuliser (a tremor in hospitalised patients has been
a common sign of nebulisers!)
 D **False**   this is simply a vasodilator effect, beta-antagonists
are absolutely contraindicated (bronchoconstriction).
 E **False**   phentolamine is an alpha-antagonist

5.14 A **False**   delays premature labour
 B **True**   stimulates uterine contraction
 C **False**   dangerous rubbish
 D **True**   older treatment, oestrogen, risked thromboembolism
 E **True**   atenolol, oxprenolol and hydralazine are also safe

5.15 A **True**   a vasodilator acting via calcium (slow channel)
blockade
 B **False**   causes bradycardia like almost all beta-blockers. The
exception is pindolol, which may occasionally
increase pulse rate because of its intrinsic
sympathomimetic activity (partial agonist activity)
 C **False**   this drug is a competitive aldosterone antagonist
often used as a diuretic
 D **False**   although relaxing arteriolar smooth muscle
tachycardia is not observed with thiazide diuretics
 E **True**   a powerful vasodilator thought to act directly on
arteriolar smooth muscle

5.16 A **False**
 B **True**   via severe hypokalaemia
 C **False**   this drug is a non-absorbed antidiarrhoeal, therefore
cannot cause systemic side-effects
 D **False**
 E **True**   one of the most notorious corticosteroids in this
respect when taken systemically

5.17 A **False**   rubbish
 B **False**   has been used in the treatment of status epileptics
 C **True**   especially in myoclonus of Creutzfeld-Jacob disease
 D **False**   do not confuse with tricyclic antidepressants
 E **True**   all benzodiazepines may do so, particularly as the
dose is increased

**5.18   Parkinsonism may be a side-effect of**
    A   long-term treatment with benzhexol
    B   intramuscular fluphenazineundecanoate
    C   ethosuximide
    D   droperidol
    E   long-term debrisoquine treatment

**5.19   In a 55-year-old man prescribed digoxin for long-term congestive heart failure**
    A   the drug would have been prescribed to treat congestive heart failure
    B   digoxin could cause gynaecomastia
    C   depression of the ST segment of the e.c.g. in leads V4–V6 suggests that the drug should be stopped
    D   the occurence of xanthopsia suggests that serum digoxin concentration should be measured
    E   prescription of potassium supplements is mandatory

**5.20   The following drugs may be usefully prescribed for a patient who has a recent history of transient cerebral ischaemic episodes due to emboli from a carotid bifurcation plaque**
    A   indomethacin
    B   sulphinpyrazone
    C   chenodeoxycholic acid
    D   phenelzine
    E   dipyridamole

5.18 A **False**   anticholinergic drugs such as benzhexol are used to treat Parkinsonism

B **True**   a depot phenothiazine for schizophrenia. True of all phenothiazines and butyrophenones

C **False**   this is an anticonvulsant

D **True**   a butyropherone, like haloperidol

E **False**   prevents noradrenaline release from noradrenergic nerve terminals and has no effect on cholinergic or dopaminergic systems

5.19 A **False**   in Britain digoxin is only given for atrial fibrillation

B **True**

C **False**   inverted 'correction mark' depression in leads with dominant R wave is a digoxin-effect (but its occurence in all leads could be an early sign of toxicity)

D **True**   green-yellow vision is a side-effect and could represent toxicity

E **False**   only mandatory when a diuretic is given also

5.20 A **False**   but aspirin another prostaglandin synthetase (cyclo-oxygenase) inhibitor could be

B **True**   inhibits platelet aggregation and is uricosuric

C **False**

D **False**

E **True**   inhibits platelet aggregation, powerful vasodilator. This is now controversial

# Chapter 6

**6.1** You diagnose a urinary tract infection in a woman aged 25 years. There is no previous history of urinary infection; after taking a urine sample for culture it would be appropriate to choose which of the following oral treatments?

A  gentamicin
B  amoxycillin
C  cotrimoxazole
D  vancomycin
E  nitrofurantoin (furadantin)

**6.2** Spironolactone

A  antagonises the action of aldosterone
B  increases potassium excretion
C  worsens glucose control in diabetes mellitus
D  can be used to treat hypertension
E  accelerates healing of gastric ulcers

**6.3** In a patient with Crohn's disease

A  sulphasalazine (salazopyrine) is useful in preventing relapses
B  diarrhoea can be alleviated by cholestyramine
C  oral sodium cromoglycate is beneficial
D  desferrioxamine is useful to treat acute attacks
E  metronidazole may heal perianal fistulae

**6.4** In a patient with radiolucent gallstones

A  chenodeoxycholate may be curative
B  ursodeoxycholate treatment may cause gallstone calcification
C  medical treatment should be continued for at least 6 months if an opaque stone is found at the ampulla of Vater
D  a low cholesterol diet may be helpful
E  alpha-hydroxycholecaliferol (hydroxy-vitamin D) would encourage gallstone dissolution

6.1  A **False**     should be reserved for serious infections and can only be given parenterally

   B **True**      well excreted in urine but some forms of *E. coli* may be resistant to amoxycillin

   C **True**      trimethoprim alone is as effective as the combination with sulphamethoxazole in cotrimoxazole

   D **False**     not absorbed from gut and is toxic when given parenterally. Vancomycin is used for *Clostridium difficile*, the organism in pseudomembranous colitis

   E **False**     reserved for resistant strains or prophlylaxis of repeated infections

6.2  A **True**      a competitive antagonist

   B **False**     retains potassium, cf. aldosterone which retains sodium and causes potassium loss

   C **False**     thiazides and loop diuretics (and also beta-blockers) have this effect. Spironolactone is useful instead of thiazides in hypertension in diabetics

   D **True**

   E **False**     it interferes with the healing of gastric ulcers by carbenoxolone

6.3  A **True**      also in ulcerative colitis

   B **True**      terminal ileitis prevents bile salt absorption resulting in bile salt colitis; cholestyramine binds bile salts

   C **False**     cromoglycate is useful in food allergy; its use in ulcerative colitis is debatable, it is useless in Crohn's

   D **False**     rubbish

   E **True**      mechanism unknown but possibly related to its activity against anaerobic bacteria

6.4  A **True**      may need treatment for at least 1 year, stones should be less than 15 mm diameter

   B **True**      a side-effect of dissolution with ursodeoxycholate, a newly-marketed alternative to chenodeoxycholate

   C **False**     because the stone is at the ampulla of Vater. The patient would be in danger of acute pancreatitis, the stone should be urgently removed. Calcified gallstones never respond to bile salts or bile acids.

   D **True**      in combination with cheno- or ursodeoxycholate

   E **False**     this drug is used only in vitamin D-resistant states when 1-hydroxylation of vitamin $D_3$ (cholecalciferol) is deficient

**6.5**   **'Physiological' neonatal jaundice may be of severe degree and may cause kernicterus; it may be**

A   reduced by treating the mother with phenobarbitone before parturition
B   reduced by treating the mother with dexamethasone before parturition
C   reduced by treating the infant with near-ultra-violet light
D   reduced by treating the infant with chenodeoxycholic acid
E   reduced by treating the mother with rifampicin before parturition

**6.6**   **In a patient with myasthenia gravis**

A   corticosteroid treatment for the myasthenia may be started in outpatients and adjusted according to response
B   sudden worsening may be provoked by gentamicin
C   sudden worsening may be provoked by beta-antagonists
D   thymectomy may be of benefit
E   pralidoxime is a useful adjunct to treatment with pyridostigmine

**6.7**   **Orthostatic (postural) hypotension may be an important adverse effect of**

A   hydralazine
B   prazosin
C   propranolol
D   imipramine
E   L-dopa (levodopa)

**6.8**   **In a patient with Parkinson's disease**

A   L-dopa relieves tremor better than rigidity
B   carbidopa decreases the risk of nausea when combined with L-dopa
C   benzhexol (artane) relieves the tremor better than rigidity
D   pretreatment with monoamine oxidase inhibitors may enhance the response to L-dopa
E   after two years treatment with L-dopa the 'on-off' effect may occur

6.5   A **True**      by induction of liver glucuronyl transferase
      B **False**     dexamethasone preparturition enhances pulmonary
                      surfactant synthesis
      C **True**      blue light breaks down bilirubin in the skin
      D **False**
      E **False**     rifampicin induces liver hydroxylase enzymes, not
                      glucuronyl transferase; rifampicin given to the
                      mother increases risk of neonatal haemorrhage

6.6   A **False**     initiation of steroid therapy may precipitate a
                      myasthenic crisis and must be done as an inpatient
      B **True**      all aminoglycosides are neuromuscular blockers
      C **False**     in myasthenia the defect is at neuromuscular
                      junction acetylcholine receptors; beta-antagonists
                      have no effect on these receptors
      D **True**      young male patients seem more likely to benefit
      E **False**     pralidoxime is a cholinesterase reactivator used for
                      organophosphate poisons which bind to the enzyme
                      active site, it could be used to treat pyridostigmine
                      overdosage in cholinergic crisis

6.7   A **False**
      B **True**      this seems to occur especially after the first dose
                      (jargon 'a first-dose phenomenon'), but can be
                      avoided sometimes by starting with a small dose and
                      increasing slowly
      C **False**     not seen with beta-antagonists
      D **True**      all tricyclics may cause postural hypotension
                      possibly by depleting sympathetic nerves of
                      noradrenaline for tricyclics block monoamine uptake
      E **True**      mechanism may be partly central but could also
                      involve stimulation of peripheral vasodilatory
                      dopamine receptors

6.8   A **False**     L-dopa is better for rigidity and hypokinesia
      B **True**      carbidopa or benserazide inhibit peripheral
                      conversion of levodopa to dopamine so decreasing
                      nausea and cardiac arrhythmias
      C **True**      often combined with levodopa
      D **False**     monoamine oxidase inhibitors must be withdrawn at
                      least 14 days, preferably 28, before levodopa is given
                      because of the risk of severe hypertension
                      (conversion to dopamine and noradrenaline of L-
                      dopa in the periphery with inability to break these
                      down due to monoamine oxidase inhibition)
      E **True**      this is true tolerance. This can be helped by stopping
                      levodopa for a time ('drug holiday') or using
                      bromocriptine in place of levodopa or by giving
                      levodopa doses at shorter time intervals (3 or 2 hours
                      between doses)

**6.9**  A patient is admitted with acute pulmonary oedema due to left ventricular failure blood pressure is 140/95, there is sinus tachycardia of 110; the following treatment will be of benefit

  A   supine position with legs elevated
  B   intravenous diamorphine (heroin)
  C   intravenous propranolol to slow the tachycardia
  D   loading dose of digoxin intravenously
  E   100% oxygen

**6.10**  Glaucoma may be a side-effect of the following

  A   a six months course of ethambutol
  B   oral acetazolamide
  C   enteric coated prednisolone
  D   cyclopentolate (mydrilate) eyedrops
  E   oral timolol maleate

**6.11**  Diarrhoea may be a troublesome side-effect of treatment with

  A   aluminium hydroxide for peptic ulceration
  B   guanethidine sulphate for hypertension
  C   long term use of pentazocine hydrochloride
  D   ampicillin
  E   colchicine in treatment of gout

**6.12**  Healing of gastric ulcers may be accelerated by

  A   sucrose octasulphate (sucralfate)
  B   magnesium sulphate in high dose
  C   cimetidine
  D   high-dose prednisolone
  E   fluphenazine undecanoate

**6.13**  Parkinsonian features may be precipitated by the following drugs

  A   fluphenazine undecanoate
  B   phenazocine
  C   droperidol
  D   amitriptyline
  E   high-dose metoclopramide

6.9    A **False**    patient is not hypotensive; sitting upright will help
                      the dyspnoea
       B **True**     diamorphine may act by causing pulmonary
                      vasodilatation
       C **False**    the sinus tachycardia is physiological, propranolol
                      will worsen the left ventricular function
       D **False**    digoxin offers no clear benefit in patients without
                      atrial fibrillation
       E **True**     improves the hypoxaemia and helps overcome the
                      swing to anaerobic metabolism and acidosis due to
                      poor tissue perfusion

6.10   A **False**    ethambutol causes retinal damage, not glaucoma
       B **False**    acetazolamide lowers intraocular pressure by
                      decreasing aqueous humor formation
       C **True**     corticosteroids raise intraocular pressure
       D **True**     all mydriatics can precipitate glaucoma (closed
                      angle) in patients with a susceptibility (shallow
                      anterior chamber, family history)
       E **False**    systemic and topical (eye drops) beta-antagonists
                      lower intraocular pressure

6.11   A **False**    aluminium and calcium salts are constipating
                      whereas magnesium salts tend to cause diarrhoea
       B **True**     explosive diarrhoea is a problem with adrenergic
                      neurone blockers. They are seldom used now
       C **False**    pentazocine is an opiate which tends to constipate
       D **True**     just like any broad-spectrum antibiotic
       E **True**     profuse diarrhoea (or vomiting) may limit the dose
                      which can be used

6.12   A **True**     sucralfate coats the ulcer rather like colloidal bismuth
                      (De-Nol), which also heals ulcers
       B **False**    this is a purgative not an antacid
       C **True**     so does ranitidine the other $H_2$-antagonist available
                      for prescription in Britain
       D **False**    exacerbates ulcers
       E **False**    fluphenazine undecanoate is an oily depot
                      phenothiazine preparation for schizophrenia

6.13   A **True**     all phenothiazines may
       B **False**
       C **True**     caused by all butyrophenones
       D **False**    parkinsonian patients get depressed and may need a
                      tricyclic which will not adversely affect their
                      parkinsonism
       E **True**     but tardive dyskinesias are the main movement
                      disorders encountered with metoclopramide

**6.14    Alpha-methyldopa may produce the following problems in treatment of hypertension in pregnancy**

A    drowsiness in the mother
B    hypotonia, poor sucking reflex and failure to thrive after parturition in the breast-fed infant
C    a Coombs-positive haemolytic anaemia in the mother
D    depression in the mother
E    extrapyramidal movement disorders

**6.15    A previously well 68-year-old lady taking indomethacin for knee osteoarthritis develops shortness of breath, ankle oedema and raised jugular venous pressure; she is in sinus rhythm. The following are true**

A    she is in heart failure
B    fluid retention by indomethacin may have caused these new features
C    combination of a beta-blocker with this drug is indicated in this patient
D    treatment with digoxin is indicated
E    indomethacin should be replaced by ibuprofen (brufen)

**6.16    A 25-year-old lady 26 weeks pregnant develops glycosuria, thirst, polyuria, pruritis vulvae and raised blood glucose concentration. The following are true**

A    If she is treated with insulin, a monocomponent, highly purified insulin may be better than a traditional insulin
B    glibenclamide is a useful alternative to insulin if she dislikes injections
C    if insulin treatment is chosen, admission to hospital and stabilisation of insulin treatment is not necessary until 38 weeks of pregnancy
D    the dose of insulin is best adjusted according to the urine glucose concentration
E    clotrimazole (canesten) may be appropriate treatment for pruritis vulvae until culture results become available

**6.17    A young lactating mother is found to be hypertensive. The following management is correct**

A    lactation should be immediately stopped with diethyl stilboestrol
B    captopril (capoten) is the drug of choice for treatment of the hypertension
C    methyldopa would not be secreted in the breast milk if methyldopa was given to the mother
D    her blood pressure may increase further during breast-feeding
E    urinary vanillyl mandelic acid excretion (VMA) should be measured as part of her management

6.14  A **True**    a common side-effect of methyldopa
      B **False**   this 'floppy infant syndrome' is produced by
                    maternal benzodiazepine ingestion
      C **True**    can occur with or without pregnancy
      D **True**    must always be watched for with methyldopa
      E **False**

6.15  A **True**
      B **True**    indomethacin causes sodium and water retention
      C **False**   beta-blockade would worsen the failure.
      D **False**   she is in sinus rhythm so that digoxin is not needed,
                    stopping the indomethacin may be all that is needed
      E **False**   ibuprofen is a non-steroidal anti-inflammatory drug
                    like indomethacin and may also cause fluid retention

6.16  A **True**    there is probably less likelihood of insulin antibodies
                    with highly purified insulins, insulin antibodies cross
                    the placenta and cause fetal hyperinsulinaemia
      B **False**   insulin is needed because sulphonylureas cross the
                    placenta and may cause fetal hypoglycaemia
      C **False**   immediate admission to hospital and stabilisation on
                    insulin is needed; after this, routine admission from
                    32 weeks to term is needed because of the risk of late
                    complications
      D **False**   in any diabetic blood glucose concentrations are
                    needed for accurate dose adjustment — remember
                    too the low renal glucose threshold of pregnancy
      E **True**    candidiasis is likely — this and thirst/polyuria will
                    also disappear after insulin treatment

6.17  A **False**   there is no need to stop lactation and
                    diethylstilboestrol would be the wrong drug to use
                    (risk of thromboembolism); bromocriptine is
                    preferable
      B **False**   captopril is a new drug and could not be given with
                    confidence in case of breast milk secretion of the
                    captopril
      C **True**    methyldopa is safe and will not be passed to the
                    baby in milk
      D **True**    the surge of prolactin and oxytocin secretion
                    provoked by the suckling reflex increases blood
                    pressure
      E **True**    the mother is young and secondary causes of
                    hypertension should be sought in any young patient

**6.18    The Committee on Safety of Medicines (CSM)**

A    considers the data on new drugs to decide if they are safe for investigation in patients

B    are funded by the Association of the British Pharmaceutical Industry

C    may recommend that a product licence be granted by the DHSS to allow a company to market a drug for a specific condition

D    collects records of all prescriptions of new drugs made by hospital and general practitioners in the NHS

E    may be informed of an adverse reaction to a drug by the yellow card system

**6.19    A young lady of 25 years of age presents with exophthalmos, sinus tachycardia and goitre; her serum thyroxine is elevated and thyroid stimulating hormone (TSH) is decreased. The following are true in relation to this lady**

A    her hyperthyroidism is likely to be primary

B    she should be treated with radioactive iodine

C    the size of the goitre will increase if she receives carbimazole

D    oral iodine should be given prior to operation if a thyroidectomy is indicated

E    beta-blocker treatment is contraindicated for she may require thyroidectomy

**6.20    A 30-year-old schizophrenic man is treated with fluphenazine decanoate injections once every three weeks, oral chlorpromazine nightly and diazepam twice daily for anxiety. He has no schizophreniform disturbance but has fainting attacks on standing associated with a fall in blood pressure, poverty of facial movement, a tremor, rigidity of both arms and difficulty in dressing**

A    he needs to be given his fluphenazine a week earlier

B    addition of benzhexol to his treatment would alleviate the tremor

C    phenylephrine (an alpha-agonist) must be given to treat his postural hypotension

D    the same treatment should be continued and he should be advised to use zips instead of buttons on his clothes

E    if he develops jaundice the fluphenazine must be stopped

6.18 A **False**    all pharmacological and toxicological and normal
human subject data must be presented for review
before a clinical trial certificate is granted to allow
investigation in large numbers of patients, a clinical
trial exemption certificate may be granted quicker, on
the basis of less data, for trials in a small number
(20–30) of patients for no more than 28 days
continual dosing of the drug. This is not done by the
CSM but by the Medicines Division of the DHSS

    B **False**    the CSM is completely independent of the ABPI
    C **True**    if the drug is safe and efficacious
    D **False**    there is no satisfactory system for this
    E **True**    an important (sadly oft-neglected) duty of doctors is
to report adverse reactions via 'yellow cards'

6.19 A **True**    increased thyroxine output inhibits pituitary TSH
secretion
    B **False**    she is not menopausal!
    C **True**    initial increased size is common — beware
retrostenal goitres
    D **True**    iodine decreases gland vascularity
    E **False**    beta-blockade reduces and is not usually a
preoperative problem but prevents 'thyroid storm'
post-thyroidectomy (look this up)

6.20 A **False**    the injection should be delayed: his schizophrenia is
controlled and he has phenothiazine side-effects
    B **True**    benzhexol alleviates parkinsonian tremor
    C **False**    the alpha-blocking action of fluphenazine and
chlopromazine may be the cause of the hypotension
— decreasing the dose or stopping these drugs is
indicated
    D **False**
    E **True**    cholestatic jaundice must be watched for with depot
phenothiazines

# Chapter 7

## 7.1 The ABPI Data Sheet compendium

A is compiled by the Committee on Safety of Medicines

B is a collection of data sheets for drugs made by pharmaceutical companies which are members of the Association of British Pharmaceutical Industry

C is distributed to doctors free of charge by the Department of Health and Social Security

D is published annually

E gives an assessment, made by an independent committee of experts, on the efficacy and safety of drugs made by pharmaceutical companies

## 7.2 The efficacy of a drug

A can be demonstrated in a double blind trial comparing the drug with a placebo

B is greater for drug A if A is effective in a dose of 100 micrograms than for drug B if B is effective in a dose of 100 milligrams

C is a measure of the bioavailability of a drug

D is a measure of the amount of a drug required to produce a given effect or action

E describes the ability of a drug to produce its therapeutic effect

## 7.3 In juvenile rheumatoid arthritis (Still's disease)

A rheumatoid factor can never be identified in the blood

B high doses of systemic corticosteroids are the treatment of choice

C physiotherapy is important in the management of children suffering from this disease

D ibuprofen or naproxen can be effective treatment

E the prognosis is good with most children reaching adulthood with no residual disability

7.1 A **False**    the CSM have nothing to do with the ABPI
                   compendium
    B **True**
    C **False**
    D **True**     it is an annual update by pharmaceutical companies
                   of the data sheets approved for their products by the
                   Medicines Division of the DHSS
    E **False**    each data sheet is the sole responsibility of each
                   pharmaceutical company and so cannot be impartial

7.2 A **True**     for most drugs this is needed to show efficacy;
                   exceptions on grounds of ethics are oral
                   contraceptives, antibiotics for life-threatening
                   infections
    B **False**    drug A is simply more *potent* than drug B
    C **False**
    D **False**    this is the potency of a drug; it is not necessarily
                   related to the efficacy of a drug. For example,
                   bumetamide 0.5 mg may produce a diuresis in a
                   patient with cardiac failure who would require
                   frusemide 20 mg to produce a similar diuresis; this
                   means that bumetamide is more potent than
                   frusemide but not that it is a better diuretic
    E **True**     it is measured as the maximum effect possible, e.g.
                   the maximum analgesic effect of morphine is greater
                   than that of aspirin

7.3 A **False**    rheumatoid factor is always present
    B **False**    corticosteroids, because of their effects on growth
                   and other side-effects, should be avoided wherever
                   possible
    C **True**     the parents have an important role here
    D **True**     paediatric suspensions of both are available
    E **True**

**7.4    Alcohol**

A    undergoes hepatic metabolism to acetaldehyde and acetate
B    may precipitate fits in epileptic patients previously stabilised on phenytoin
C    decreases the hypnotic effect of nitrazepam
D    causes flushing, vomiting, tachycardia and headache if ingested by a patient taking disulfiram
E    inhibits the hypoglycaemic effect of chlorpropamide

**7.5    Under the Medicines Act (1968) in the United Kingdom**

A    a new drug may be tested by a pharmaceutical company in up to 20 patients without formal permission from the Department of Health and Social Security
B    the drug can be marketed by a pharmaceutical company only if a product licence application to the DHSS is successful
C    the Committee on Review of Medicines (CRM) scrutinises the applications from parmaceutical companies who wish to market new drugs in the UK
D    a new drug may be tested on any number of normal subjects without formal permission from the DHSS
E    large scale trials of a new drug in patients can be carried out if a clinical trial certificate is granted for the drug

**7.6    Acyclovir is**

A    a cyclic aminoglycoside antibiotic
B    effective treatment for herpes simplex encephalitis
C    may prevent the blisters of herpes labialis if given during the prodrome preceding cold sore development
D    is active orally in the prophylaxis of primary infection by herpes simplex type II (genital herpes) virus
E    gives rise to an active metabolite which inhibits viral DNA polymerase

**7.7    A patient with left ventricular failure develops pulmonary oedema, the following could be logical components of his treatment**

A    intravenous diamorphine (heroin)
B    intravenous potassium chloride
C    intravenous digoxin to increase left ventricular output
D    intravenous dobutamine would decrease afterload by blocking alpha-adrenoceptors in the resistance vessels
E    intravenous dopamine would decrease afterload by blocking alpha-adrenoceptors in the resistance vessels

7.4  A **True**
    B **True**    alcohol itself is epileptogenic but it also induces hepatic enzymes — both actions may decrease the effectiveness of anticonvulsants
    C **False**    alcohol potentiates all sedatives
    D **True**    the 'antabuse reaction' — due to inhibition of acetaldehyde dehydrogenase with build-up of acetaldehyde
    E **False**    alcohol stimulates insulin release and so is hypoglycaemic in its own right: always check blood glucose in acute alcohol intoxicants admitted to hospital

7.5  A **False**    before a new drug can be given to any patients the company must be granted by the DHSS a clinical trial certificate (CTC) or exemption from holding a clinical trial certificate (CTX scheme)
    B **True**    a product licence application is scrutinised by the Committee on Safety of Medicines who make a recommendation to the Medicines Division of the DHSS; the Medicines Division then decide whether to grant the licence
    C **False**    the CRM only reviews 'older' medicines which were given product licences before the Medicines Act came into effect in 1971. The CRM does not deal with applications for licences for new drugs
    D **True**    unlike the situation in the USA where FDA permission must first be obtained
    E **True**

7.6  A **False**
    B **True**    given by intravenous infusion it is better than cytosine arabinoside
    C **True**
    D **False**    but given orally or intravenously it can accelerate healing of genital ulcers after infection
    E **True**    viral thymidine kinase converts acyclovir to the triphosphate which then inhibits viral DNA synthesis by inhibiting viral DNA polymerase

7.7  A **True**
    B **False**    intravenous potassium chloride is dangerous and can cause fatal cardiac arrhythmias it must be used very *cautiously*
    C **False**    intravenous digoxin is dangerous and only needed for atrial fibrillation
    D **False**    dobutamine is a beta$_1$-selective inotrope
    E **False**    dopamine stimulates alpha-receptors at high doses

**7.8    In a patient with septicaemia due to *Pseudomonas aeruginosa***

A    treatment of choice would be intravenous high-dose ampicillin

B    intravenous gentamicin would be effective treatment

C    tobramycin and amikacin could cause eighth cranial nerve deafness

D    measurement of plasma concentrations of gentamicin would be an unnecessary investigation if this drug were used

E    an aminoglycoside would synergise with a beta-lactam antibiotic

**7.9    Which of the following drugs are recognised for treatment of raised intraocular pressure**

A    high-dose intravenous frusemide

B    topical timolol eye drops

C    oral acetazalomide

D    corticosteroid eye drops

E    oral bendrofluazide

**7.10    Glaucoma, a damaging increase of intraocular pressure, may occur as a side-effect of**

A    corticosteroid eye drops

B    oral corticosteroid treatment

C    oral indomethacin

D    chloramphenicol eye ointment

E    homatropine eye drops

**7.11    The following drugs are known to be harmful to the fetus if given to the mother during pregnancy**

A    aldomet (alpha-methyldopa)

B    prednisolone

C    ethanol

D    oxprenolol

E    warfarin

**7.12    In a patient with hypertension and chronic renal failure**

A    combined treatment with captopril and spironolactone may cause potassium depletion

B    treatment of osteoarthritis with flurbiprofen may worsen the hypertension

C    high doses of guanethidine are safe for treating the hypertension

D    combined treatment with propranolol and spironolactone may cause increased Twave and decreased Rwave heights in the e.c.g.

E    combined treatment with captopril and bendrofluazide may be hazardous

7.8    A **False**
       B **True**
       C **True**    both drugs, like all aminoglycosides, cause eighth
                     nerve deafness, vestibular damage
       D **False**   plasma concentration measurements are mandatory
                     for safe effective therapy
       E **True**    examples are tobramycin or gentamycin plus
                     carbenicillin. The new cephalosporin ceftazidime may
                     be effective alone against *Pseudomonas*

7.9    A **False**
       B **True**    other beta-antagonist eye drops are used for
                     glaucoma
       C **True**    decreases formation of aqueous humor by inhibiting
                     carbonic anhydrase
       D **False**   but plausible, eh?
       E **False**

7.10   A **True**
       B **True**
       C **False**
       D **False**
       E **True**    contraction of ciliary muscle dilates the pupil and
                     blocks the aqueous humour drainage canal

7.11   A **False**   safe for hypertension of pregnancy
       B **True**    cleft-palate described
       C **True**    decreased birth-weight
       D **False**   safe for hypertension in pregnancy
       E **True**    cleft palate

7.12   A **False**   angiotensin converting enzyme inhibition (decreased
                     aldosterone synthesis) by captopril and aldosterone
                     antagonism by spironolactone cause hyperkalaemia;
                     this combination could be contraindicated
       B **True**    non-steroidal anti-inflammatory drugs cause sodium
                     retention and worsen hypertension
       C **False**   renal clearance of guanethidine is decreased so
                     dangerous hypotension may result
       D **True**    both drugs cause potassium retention;
                     hyperkalaemia causes these e.c.g. changes. Obscure
                     question!
       E **True**    this combination is reported to cause reversible renal
                     failure

**7.13 In a patient with chronic paraplegia**

A weekly intramuscular gentamicin is good prophylaxis against urinary tract infection

B baclofen is useful in preventing flexor spasms

C diazepam may be given to decrease spasticity

D chronic nitrofurantoin treatment may cause a peripheral neuropathy

E noxythiolin (noxyflex) is useful to treat urinary infections if the patient has an indwelling urinary catheter

**7.14 The following are true of a female patient with epilepsy**

A if she becomes pregnant the epilepsy may worsen

B if she becomes pregnant her treatment with phenytoin should be stopped for the first trimester because of the risk of teratogenesis

C if she is young and still at school, phenytoin is preferable to carbamazepine because of the drowsiness associated with carbamazepine treatment

D if her fits occur at the time of her periods she should be given an oral contraceptive which may decrease the fit frequency

E if she is schizophrenic and treated with fluphenazine undecanoate (a phenothiazine) her fit frequency may increase

**7.15 In a male patient with psoriasis**

A exposure to ultraviolet light will worsen the disease

B treatment with dithranol may burn the skin

C Whitfield's ointment is a recognised treatment

D methoxypsoralen can be a helpful treatment

E methotrexate is useful in resistant cases

7.13 A **False**  this important drug should be reserved for severe infections with organisms resistant to other antibiotics

   B **True**  baclofen is a gamma-aminobutyric acid (GABA) agonist, GABA inhibits spinal reflexes

   C **True**  benzodiazepine receptors are intimately linked with GABA receptors and chloride ion channels; this probably accounts for the antispastic action of benzodiazepines

   D **True**  nitrofurantoin is sometimes used for prophylaxis of urinary tract infections

   E **True**  a urinary 'antiseptic' useful for mixed growths and instilled into the bladder via the catheter

7.14 A **True**  it is often said that pregnancy makes epilepsy worse, but there is evidence in animals that makes this belief debatable

   B **False**  epilepsy itself seems to be associated with a slightly increased risk of congenital deformities. However, anticonvulsants must be continued; blood levels should be measured so as to use the minimum dose possible

   C **False**  the reverse is true: carbamazepine does not impair alertness (in therapeutic doses) but phenytoin and phenobarbitone often do

   D **False**  rubbish. The pill may worsen epilepsy. Catamenial epilepsy (fits around the periods) can be treated with usual anticonvulsants

   E **True**  phenothiazines may worsen epilepsy

7.15 A **False**  ultraviolet A (PUVA) helps to clear quite severe lesions; sunlight has been known to be beneficial for many years. However, PUVA is associated with increased risk of skin neoplasms

   B **True**  dithranol in Lasser's paste is a good treatment, but if too strong a concentration is used or if the dithranol touches normal skin burning may occur — put paraffin wax around the lesions to stop the dithranol getting onto normal skin

   C **False**  Whitfield's ointment is antifungal

   D **True**  enters the skin and absorbs u.v. light, so augmenting PUVA

   E **True**  it interferes with gametogenesis and is hepatotoxic, so is a last resort

**7.16  In acne rosacea**

A   topical dithranol cures the skin lesions
B   oral tetracyclines may improve the condition
C   ungentum cocois co. (coconut oil ointment) may improve scalp manifestations
D   there is an increased risk of underlying visceral malignancy
E   systemic corticosteroids are the treatment of choice

**7.17  In a patient with Hodgkin's disease diagnosed as at stage I**

A   treatment will need to be life long
B   no treatment is needed unless symptoms develop
C   flushing may occur if the patient takes alcohol
D   the treatment of choice is local radiotherapy
E   treatment results in about 80% patients surviving for 5 years after diagnosis

**7.18  A male patient may complain of erectile impotence and/or failure of ejaculation due to treatment with the following drugs**

A   nitrazepam
B   hydralazine
C   aspirin
D   debrisoquine
E   a thiazide diuretic

**7.19  In a patient taking digoxin and hydrochlorthiazide the following side-effects may be due to one or both drugs**

A   precipitation of asthma
B   worsening of acne vulgaris
C   xanthopsia (green or yellow vision)
D   pulsus bigeminus
E   glycosuria

**7.20  The following side-effects of drugs are dose-related (occur with higher doses of the drugs)**

A   hypokalaemia on bendrofluazide
B   precipitation of asthma by aspirin
C   impaired glucose tolerance by thiazide diuretics
D   haemolytic anaemia with alpha-methyldopa
E   nephrotoxicity of lithium

7.16 A **False**
    B **True**
    C **True**     applied at night (messy!) and removed with coal tar shampoo
    D **False**    do not confuse with increased incidence in squamous carcinoma of the skin and acanthosis nigricans
    E **False**

7.17 A **False**
    B **False**    rubbish. The disease may first be noticed as an enlarged single lymph node but investigation and treatment should be immediate
    C **True**     mechanism unknown
    D **True**     to the the area which will be localised to one side of the diaphragm — laparotomy is needed for staging
    E **True**     there is a good chance of cure

7.18 A **False**    benzodiazepines do not cause impotence
    B **False**
    C **False**
    D **True**     all the adrenergic neurone blocking drugs may cause this
    E **True**     so too may beta-antagonists and alpha-antagonists.

7.19 A **False**    neither drug is known to precipitate asthma
    B **False**
    C **True**     a sign of digoxin intoxication
    D **True**     cardiac arrhythmia classically associated with digoxin
    E **True**     diabetogenic effect of thiazides

7.20 A **True**     the risk can be lessened by keeping the dose low because the antihypertensive effect of thiazides is 'saturable' and does not increase linearly with dose
    B **False**    allergic phenomenon — Samter triad = nasal polyps, hay fever and asthma precipitated by aspirin
    C **True**
    D **False**    an 'allergic' phenomenon
    E **True**     plasma level measurement is mandatory to keep lithium concentrations within the therapeutic range

# Chapter 8

**8.1** A rectal temperature of below 35°C (accidental hypothermia) may be caused in elderly patients by the following drugs

    **A**   chlorpromazine
    **B**   thioridazine
    **C**   bendrofluazide
    **D**   ethanol
    **E**   chlorpropamide

**8.2** A 72-year-old patient complains of dizziness on standing, which is associated with a blood pressure of 86/48 compared with a pressure of 136/94 on lying supine (phase V diastolic). The following drugs may have caused this

    **A**   diazepam
    **B**   amitriptyline
    **C**   chlorpromazine
    **D**   alpha-methyldopa
    **E**   pindolol

**8.3** A patient with disseminated sclerosis complains of painful flexor muscle spasms and on examination is shown to have marked increased tone in the legs (spasticity). The following drugs may help this patient

    **A**   L-dopa combined with a decarboxylase inhibitor
    **B**   diazepam
    **C**   baclofen
    **D**   chlorpromazine
    **E**   haloperidol

**8.4** A patient presents with recent onset of writhing facial movements (orofacial, tardive, dyskinesia). The following drugs are known as a possible cause of this condition

    **A**   cimetidine
    **B**   L-dopa combined with a decarboxylase inhibitor
    **C**   metoclopramide
    **D**   haloperidol
    **E**   an injection one week previously of modecate (an oily depot injection of thioridazine, a phenothiazine)

8.1   A **True**    inhibits hypothalamic thermoregulation
      B **True**    a phenothiazine commonly used as melleril to treat
                    elderly confusion — CARE!
      C **False**
      D **True**    a common cause, also in young drunken subjects
      E **False**   although unconsciousness from hypoglycaemia
                    could feasibly cause hypothermia

8.2   A **False**   postural hypotension is not caused by
                    benzodiazepines in humans (but does occur with
                    large intravenous doses in animals)
      B **True**    the patient has postural hypotension. Mianserin is
                    said to produce less postural hypotension than
                    amitriptyline and other tricyclic antidepressants
      C **True**    chlorpromazine and all phenothiazines are alpha-
                    adrenoceptor blockers.
      D **True**    you must always be aware of this: many older
                    hypertensives will be taking this drug
      E **False**   postural hypotension is not caused by beta-
                    adrenoceptor antagonists

8.3   A **False**   L-dopa is only of use in extrapyramidal system
                    rigidity in primary idiopathic or secondary
                    parkinsonism
      B **True**    benzodiazepines inhibit spinal reflexes and so
                    decrease spasticity
      C **True**    baclofen is a gamma-amino butyric acid (GABA)
                    agonist which inhibits spinal reflexes; other GABA
                    agonists are being developed
      D **False**
      E **False**

8.4   A **False**
      B **True**    a distressing side-effect of L-dopa, combination with
                    a decarboxylase inhibitor decreases peripheral side-
                    effects (nausea, tachycardia) but not central side-
                    effects
      C **True**    metoclopramide is a dopamine antagonist
      D **True**    haloperidol and other butyrophenones are dopamine
                    antagonists
      E **True**    thioridazine is a phenothiazine, phenothiazines are
                    dopamine antagonists

**8.5    The following are true of sodium valproate (valproic acid sodium)**

A    it may be given to prevent febrile convulsions in children/infants
B    it is used to treat parkinsonism
C    it may cause disturbance of liver function tests
D    it is a beta-adrenoceptor antagonist
E    it is effective in treatment of petit mal epilepsy

**8.6    The following items were included in a single prescription by a doctor: 'sulphasalazine 500 mg t.d.s (means three times daily) for 365 days and colifoam (foam containing hydrocortisone acetate 10%) b.d (means twice daily) for 365 days'. The pharmacist would be correct in the following actions, thoughts or comments**

A    the pharmacist should dispense the drugs as requested
B    he should contact the doctor to suggest that the duration covered by the prescription is too long
C    he thinks that the patient is likely to have ulcerative colitis
D    he is correct when he asks the doctor to write 'three times' and 'twice' 'daily' instead of, respectively, 't.d.s.' and 'b.d.'
E    the doses of the drugs used and the amounts prescribed should be written in words as well as figures

**8.7    A prescription for a 'prescription-only' drug is legally invalid if**

A    it is not written on a proper hospital in- or outpatient prescription form or the orange FP10 form used by general practitioners and hospital outpatient doctors
B    if it does not contain the patient's address
C    if it is signed by a dentist but not countersigned by a registered doctor
D    it does not state the name of the parent or guardian of a child named on the prescription and said to be under 12 years old
E    if it is for morphine sulphate written as follows: 'morphine sulphate sustained release 10 mg (TEN), b.d. (TWICE). Please give 4 weeks supply'

8.5  A **True**    it is the drug of choice for this
     B **False**
     C **True**    this is not widely enough known, but now *you* know,
                   so monitor liver enzymes!
     D **False**
     E **True**    a good alternative to ethosuximide

8.6  A **False**
     B **True**    this encourages the patient not to be assessed by a
                   doctor and is unsafe. Colifoam contains a large
                   amount of topical steroid and should not be
                   prescribed continuously for a year
     C **True**
     D **True**    as recommended by the British National Formulary,
                   o.d., nocte, t.i.d., t.d.s., b.i.d., b.d., rep. mist. (repeat
                   prescription), ad lib (as needed) are OBSOLETE for
                   prescriptions
     E **False**   only needs words as well as figures and the exact
                   number of tablets/volumes to be prescribed in the
                   case of controlled drugs

8.7  A **False**   provided it has the name and address of the patient,
                   describes type, dose, duration and any other details
                   necessary for safe, legal dispensing and provided
                   that it is signed by the doctor or dentist it can be
                   written on any paper — this is common for private
                   prescriptions
     B **True**
     C **False**   dentists may prescribe from a list of certain drugs:
                   notably antibiotics and minor analgesics
     D **False**   the name and address of the child is enough
     E **True**    the exact *dose* and *number* of tablets (or volume of
                   liquid) must be written in words and figures. The
                   correct version is morphine sulphate sustained
                   release 10 mg (TEN MILLIGRAMS) TWICE DAILY FOR
                   FOUR WEEKS. Please supply 28 (twenty eight) 10 mg
                   (ten milligram) tablets

**8.8**    A patient with idiopathic parkinsonism has been treated with L-dopa for 2 years. He has found that his parkinsonian symptoms have returned about 6 hours after taking his morning dose and on rising in the morning (about 10 hours after taking his evening dose). The following statements about this patient are true:

A    he suffers from the 'on-off' phenomenon
B    his L-dopa should be given in more frequent doses than twice daily
C    if he is given bromocriptine this may help to alleviate his symptoms
D    the L-dopa is likely to benefit his parkinsonian tremor much more-than any rigidity.
E    the period of return of his parkinsonian symptoms may be caused by impaired L-dopa entry into the brain

**8.9**    The following are true with respect to drugs used in elderly patients (age arbitrarily above 65 years) relative to young adults

A    elderly patients are less sensitive to the hypnotic effects of benzodiazepines
B    renal clearance of digoxin is greater in the elderly
C    renal clearance of gentamicin is decreased in the elderly
D    atropine is preferred to scopolamine for premedication in elderly patients
E    sensitivity of the bradycardia response to beta-antagonists is greater in elderly patients

**8.10**    A patient stabilised on phenytoin for epilepsy becomes mildly depressed, is seen in outpatients and is given amitriptyline. Two days later she is seen in casualty having had a fit at 8 a.m. that morning. The following statements are true

A    the casualty officer should arrange for measurement of plasma phenytoin concentration
B    she will lose her driving licence
C    since the depression was mild, psychotherapy could be tried instead of amitriptyline
D    amitriptyline may have provoked the fit
E    a history of alcohol abuse and a recent binge might be relevant in explaining the fit

8.8   A **True**    the 'on-off' periods are, respectively, the times when
                    his parkinsonian symptoms are absent or present; it
                    is tolerance to L-dopa
      B **True**    even 2-or 3-hourly
      C **True**    bromocriptine may help with rigidity and akinesia,
                    but is often unsuccessful in the on-off phenomenon
      D **False**   anticholinergics are best for the tremor, L-dopa
                    for the rigidity and hypokinesia
      E **True**    protein meals release phenylalanine, leucine and
                    isoleucine, bulky amino acids which compete with
                    L-dopa for transport across the blood-brain barrier

8.9   A **False**   the sensitivity in terms of sleep response is the same
                    but because of decreased nervous function and with
                    some benzodiazepines, decreased body clearance,
                    elderly patients are more likely to suffer confusion,
                    day-time drowsiness and the consequences of these
                    (falls, bed sores, loss of independence — CARE!)
      B **False**   renal function decreases with age — check blood
                    digoxin concentrations!
      C **True**
      D **True**    scopolamine is more likely to cause confusion for
                    some unknown reason
      E **False**   sensitivity to bradycardia with beta-antagonists and
                    to the tachycardia response to beta-agonists is less in
                    the elderly; nevertheless take care with prescription
                    (decreased drug elimination in the elderly, impaired
                    cardiovascular reflexes)

8.10  A **True**    to check the concentration is in the therapeutic range
                    and to check compliance
      B **True**    patients must be fit-free during daytime for three
                    years before they can have a driving licence
      C **True**
      D **True**    well known for tricyclic antidepressants
      E **True**    alcohol is an enzyme inducer and could result in
                    increased phenytoin metabolism, conversely alcohol
                    intoxication or withdrawal can cause a fit

**8.11**  A patient is prescribed topical timolol eye-drops for his condition. Shortly after starting the eye drops, he has an attack of breathlessness with expiratory wheezes and a fall in peak-expiratory flow rate. The following are true

A  the patient probably had glaucoma
B  pilocarpine eye drops could have been used for this patient
C  the patient had an attack of asthma caused by the timolol
D  the breathlessness would respond to intravenous amiodarone
E  the patient's pupils would have been dilated by the timolol

**8.12**  A 70-year-old lady with hypertension treated with bendrofluazide complains of severe pain in her left hip; an X-ray shows osteoarthritis. The following points may become true during the management of her hip pain

A  colchicine would relieve the pain
B  indomethacin could be prescribed for the painful hip condition
C  if she is prescribed ibuprofen, a non-steroidal anti-inflammatory drug, her blood pressure may increase
D  oral corticosteroid treatment could be given if the hip pain was not relieved by other drugs
E  the bendrofluazide is likely to have caused the hip condition

**8.13**  The following drugs are appropriate treatment for the condition given

A  ethosuximide for petit mal
B  minoxidil for idiopathic hirsuitism
C  hydrochlorthiazide (a thiazide diuretic) for nephrogenic diabetes insipidus
D  sodium valproate for petit mal
E  cis-retinoic acid (topical) for psoriasis

**8.14**  In a double-blind, cross-over trial of a new drug A compared with an established drug B, it is true that

A  one group of patients will take only drug A and a separate group will take only drug B to the end of the trial
B  in Britain this clinical trial will need the permission of the Department of Health and Social Security
C  the doctor measuring the patients' responses to the drugs will know which treatment each patient is taking but the patients will not
D  if drug A has a long elimination half-life it may interfere initially with evaluation of the response to drug B, if drug A is given first
E  if the variables which the investigating physician is measuring are all normally distributed, then the results may be evaluated statistically using parametric statistics

8.11  A **True**
      B **True**
      C **True**    this is well-known, sufficient beta-antagonist may be
                    absorbed through the conjunctiva and presumably
                    via the nose and pharynx after draining via the
                    nasolacrymal duct
      D **False**
      E **False**   alpha-agonists dilate the pupils, not beta-antagonists

8.12  A **False**   colchicine can only relieve gouty joint pain (almost
                    diagnostic of gout)
      B **True**    non-steroidal anti-inflammatory drugs are commonly
                    used for the pain
      C **True**    be aware of this common side-effect
      D **False**
      E **False**   rubbish

8.13  A **True**
      B **False**   minoxidil causes hirsuitism
      C **True**
      D **True**    probably a better choice than ethosuximide
      E **False**   cis-retinoic acid topically is used for acne and
                    icthyosis; another retinoid etretinate is used for
                    psoriasis

8.14  A **False**   in a cross-over trial, each patient will take each drug
                    A and B in an order randomly assigned
      B **True**    a clinical trial certificate or exemption from one (CTX)
                    will be needed from the DHSS if a pharmaceutical
                    company runs the trial, but a doctor's or dentist's
                    exemption (DDX scheme) from holding a CTC or CTX
                    can be obtained by any doctor or dentist wanting to
                    initiate a trial of a new drug independently of a
                    pharmaceutical company
      C **False**   neither doctor nor patient will know ('*double*' blind).
      D **True**    this is the main criticism of cross-over trials; one is
                    never sure, especially if the first drug remains in the
                    body a long time, that it will not influence the
                    response to the second drug
      E **True**    parametric statistics can be used only for variables
                    (e.g. blood pressure) which are normally distributed,
                    the data can be statistically tested to ensure that this
                    is so; otherwise non-parametric statistics must be
                    used

Remember this.

**8.15 A withdrawal syndrome may occur when patients abruptly stop taking the following drugs**

A  diazepam for insomnia
B  propranolol for angina pectoris
C  L-dopa for idiopathic parkinsonism
D  allopurinol for idiopathic gout
E  clonidine for essential hypertension

**8.16 The following statements are correct with regard to the management of migraine**

A  ergotamine is useful for long-term treatment as prophylaxis against migraine
B  methysergide given as prophylactic may be associated with renal failure
C  pizotifen is effective as a prophylactic against migraine
D  in acute migraine, oral analgesic drug absorption may be delayed because of gastric stasis
E  in migraine patients, long-term beta-adrenoceptor antagonists are contraindicated because they may cause severe peripheral vasospasm

**8.17 In management of a patient with ascites due to liver failure**

A  spironolactone is an appropriate treatment
B  the rate of diuresis should not exceed that equivalent to a weight loss of 1 kg per day
C  the presence of hyperaldosteromism increases the risk of diuretic-induced hypokalaemia
D  use of sedative drugs may precipitate hepatic encephalopathy
E  potassium-sparing diuretics are contraindicated because of the risk of electrolyte disturbance

**8.18 The following statements are true of liver enzyme induction**

A  phenytoin given long-term increases the rate of hydroxylation by liver enzymes
B  an increase in serum gamma-glutamyl transpeptidase may be a sign of liver enzyme induction
C  an increase in serum alkaline phosphatase may be a sign of liver enzyme induction
D  if a patient on warfarin is given cimetidine the prothrombin time may be prolonged
E  liver enzyme induction may increase vitamin-D metabolism causing osteomalacia in patients taking primidone

8.15 A **True** because benzodiazepines may induce dependence
B **True** this can consist of arrhythmias, angina and even myocardial infarction: some say this is controversial, the situation being merely 'rebound' angina
C **False** the disease symptoms simply return
D **False** a gouty attack may occur
E **True** severe rebound hypertension due to excessive catecholamine secretion may occur (treat with alpha-adrenoceptor antagonist

8.16 A **False** only used in the acute attack because of the risks of ergotism
B **True** since it may cause retroperitoneal fibrosis with ureteric compression
C **True** a property shared with other 5-hydroxy tryptamine antagonists
D **True** this can be a problem also with antiemetics
E **False** beta-antagonists are recognized prophylactic treatment, those without partial agonism are the most effective

8.17 A **True** it antagonizes the sodium and water retention resulting from the hyperaldosteronism of liver failure
B **True** more rapid rates risk encephalopathy: WEIGH YOUR PATIENTS REGULARLY!
C **True**
D **True**
E **False** they are useful but plasma potassium must be checked

8.18 A **True** a good example
B **True** well established but not well-known as such: alcohol initially raises gamma GT because it is an enzyme inducer
C **True** but one must explain other causes of raised alkaline phosphatase (as for gamma GT) before assuming enzyme induction as a cause
D **True** cimetidine inhibits the liver enzymes which hydroxylate and inactivate warfarin, so the prothrombin time will be prolonged
E **True** primidone is metabolized to phenobarbitone which is a potent enzyme inducer; osteomalacia may also occur with phenytoin liver enzyme induction

**8.19  Skin reactions to drugs**

A    are much commoner after single dose than multiple dose treatment

B    may take the form of a blistering eruption after barbiturate administration

C    occur more commonly than usual when amoxycillin is given to patients with glandular fever

D    should always be treated with systemic corticosteroids in large doses

E    may occur in exactly the same site as initially if a patient who had a rash with phenolphthalein is rechallenged with this drug

**8.20  The following drugs are useful for treating fungal skin infections**

A    clotrimazole cream topically to lesions in tinea capitis or corporis

B    clotrimazole cream to affected nails in ringworm infection of the nails

C    intravenous amphotericin for severe oral candidiasis

D    topical clotrimazole for pityriasis versicolor (caused by Malassezia furfur)

E    oral griseofulvin for mucocutaneous candidiasis

8.19  A **False**
    B  **True**    'barbiturate blisters' seen in barbiturate overdoses
    C  **True**    40–50% incidence
    D  **False**    only if severe or life-threatening should systemic
              steroids be used — topically is sufficient
    E  **True**    a 'fixed drug eruption' seen with phenolphthalein,
              sulphonamides and barbiturates

8.20  A **True**    the imidazoles clotrimazole, miconazole or econazole
              are the treatments of choice (avoid ketoconazole
              since it may cause serious liver toxicity)
    B  **False**    oral griseofulvin is indicated here, topical tioconazole
              solution may be used alone or with griseofulvin
    C  **False**    *oral* amphotericin lozenges or nystatin or miconazole
              oral gel
    D  **True**    the old-fashioned Whitfield's ointment also works
    E  **False**    candida is a yeast; griseofulvin has no action against
              yeasts and is only of use against ringworm fungi

*You keep getting this wrong*

# Chapter 9

## 9.1 When a drug is given intravenously

A   a more rapid onset of effect is always achieved
B   the area under the concentration time curve will be higher than that following oral dosing for all drugs with 100% bioavailability
C   the volume of distribution will be higher
D   gastrointestinal adverse effects can be avoided
E   first pass hepatic (presystemic) metabolism does not occur

## 9.2 First pass hepatic metabolism

A   can be avoided by giving the drug via the skin
B   may be genetically determined
C   is seen when a drug has a high hepatic extraction ratio
D   is not seen when a drug is predominantly renally excreted
E   may also occur to a certain extent during the second pass through the liver

## 9.3 Frusemide

A   acts on the proximal limb of the loop of Henle
B   causes aldosterone-dependent hypokalaemia
C   has a duration of action of approximately 12 hours
D   when given i.v. in large doses should be infused in 5% dextrose
E   is active in patients with glomerular filtration rates down to 5 ml/min

## 9.4 Thiazide diuretics

A   are moderately effective carbonic anhydrase inhibitors
B   exert their hypotensive effect via a direct effect on blood vessels
C   reduce urinary calcium excretion
D   rarely cause glucose intolerance
E   are antagonised by most non-steroidal anti-inflammatory drugs

9.1  A **False**    although this is often the case, e.g. loop diuretics, it is not necessarily so, e.g. warfarin, where the drug does not have a direct effect.

    B **False**    this is only true for drugs with less than 100% bioavailability

    C **False**    rubbish — volume of distribution is independent of route of administration

    D **False**    gastrointestinal adverse effects of oral drugs are very often systemically mediated and hence will still occur after i.v.dosing

    E **True**    remember that first pass metabolism does not occur with many drugs anyway

9.2  A **True**    thus avoiding the hepatic portal circulation

    B **True**    acetylation phenotype is an important determinant of oral hydralazine pharmacokinetics

    C **True**    well demonstrated by many of the organic nitrates, e.g. GTN

    D **True**    by definition can only occur when drugs are metabolised in the liver

    E **False**    subsequent passes through the liver contribute to systemic not presystemic metabolism and have a lesser pharmacokinetic effect because distribution to the tissues has already begun

9.3  A **False**    inhibits active chloride reabsorption in the thick segment of the ascending limb of the loop

    B **True**    distal delivery of $Na^+$ produces both aldosterone-dependent and aldosterone-independent $Na^+/K^+$ exchange

    C **False**    after oral absorption it is approximately 6 hours — shorter after i.v. administration

    D **False**    difficult question — the low pH of dextrose makes saline a better choice despite the small sodium load it would contain

    E **False**    no appreciable diuretic effect below 10 ml/min

9.4  A **False**    almost all their diuretic activity is effected at the distal convoluted tubule

    B **True**    plasma volume changes are only short lived

    C **True**    note that frusemide does the opposite

    D **False**    very common

    E **True**    both diuretic and hypotensive effects are antagonised

**9.5    During warfarin therapy**

A    several days must elapse before factor IX levels reach steady state

B    loading doses enable more rapid control of prothrombin ratio

C    fixed drug eruptions may occur

D    osteoporosis may develop particularly in women

E    is useful in pregnancy because it does not cross the placenta

**9.6    In the treatment of infectious diseases**

A    high-dose i.v. penicillin is the drug of choice in suspected bacterial meningitis in adults whilst awaiting c.s.f. microscopy results

B    mithramycin should be given for *Haemophilus influenzae* epiglottitis

C    antistaphylococcal drugs are not needed in the treatment of erysipelas

D    tuberculosis can effectively be cured using only two drugs

E    erythromycin should be used routinely in the treatment of pneumonia

**9.7    Expected findings in aspirin overdosage in an adult include**

A    respiratory alkalosis

B    metabolic acidosis

C    pyrexia

D    hypokalaemia

E    coma

**9.8    Hydrochlorothiazide may be useful in the management of**

A    diabetes insipidus

B    renal calculi

C    hypertension in the elderly

D    pulmonary oedema

E    chronic bronchitis

**9.9    Treatment with methyldopa may cause**

A    weight gain

B    haemolytic anaemia

C    urinary retention

D    gynaecomastia

E    fever

9.5   A **False**   this is true of factor II (prothrombin) not factors VII, IX and X

     B **False**   this general principle of rapidly achieving steady state concentrations does not hold true here because of the long half-life of circulating prothrombin

     C **True**

     D **False**   you are thinking of heparin

     E **False**   it is associated with fetal malformations and is absolutely contraindicated in the first trimester of pregnancy

9.6   A **True**   meningococcal and pneumococcal infections are invariably the cause in adults except those with known or suspected immunodeficiency

     B **False**   this antibiotic is a cytotoxic agent to human cells as well as bacterial cells. Chloramphenicol should be given

     C **True**   this infection is always caused by streptococci which are exquisitely sensitive to penicillin

     D **False**   initial therapy must always be with three drugs e.g., rifampicin, isoniazid and ethambutol (or pyrazinamide)

     E **True**   *mycoplasma, Legionella* and *Pneumococci* are all sensitive to this drug. More recently, occasional Gram negative bacteria resistant to erythromycin has led to the combination of erythromycin and ampicillin

9.7   A **True**   often not seen in children

     B **True**   usually develops more slowly

     C **True**   like the respiratory alkalosis is due to a central stimulatory effect

     D **False**   hypokalaemia is usually due to forced alkaline diuresis

     E **False**   coma is an unusual feature

9.8   A **True**   mechanism not clear

     B **True**   if calculi contain appreciable amounts of calcium, reduction in urinary calcium will reduce stone formation

     C **True**   thiazides are drugs of choice

     D **False**   loop diuretics not thiazides are indicated

     E **False**   thiazides have no effect on sputum production

9.9   A **True**   due to fluid retention

     B **True**   rare although a positive Coomb's test alone is much more common and is dose related

     C **False**   no anticholinergic activity

     D **True**   due to hyperprolactinaemic effect

     E **True**   an unusual cause of drug fever

**9.10  Salicylate**

    A   is rapidly renally excreted in an alkaline urine
    B   potentiates the activity of warfarin
    C   is a metabolite of aspirin
    D   is uricosuric at anti-inflammatory doses
    E   has minimal antipyretic activity

**9.11  Allopurinol**

    A   may precipitate acute gout
    B   is a useful addition to 6-mercaptopurine in the treatment of myeloid leukaemia
    C   should not be used with probenecid as long-term therapy in gout
    D   can prevent the hyperuricaemia of therapeutic starvation
    E   dosage reduction is not necessary in moderately severe renal failure (GFR <30 ml/min)

**9.12  Therapy with nystatin is beneficial in**

    A   oesophageal moniliasis
    B   vaginal thrush
    C   candida septicaemia
    D   candida nail bed infection
    E   candida granuloma

**9.13  The use of corticosteroids (e.g. prednisolone 20 mg daily) may be particularly hazardous in a patient with**

    A   malignant hypertension
    B   chronic gout
    C   radiological evidence of old TB
    D   duodenal ulcer
    E   herpes zoster

**9.14  Pethidine**

    A   Causes spasm of the biliary sphincter
    B   Relaxes ureteric spasm in renal colic
    C   is less likely to cause addiction than morphine
    D   Is less likely to cause respiratory depression than morphine
    E   should be given no more often than 4-hourly

9.10  A **True**      urine flow rate is relatively unimportant compared
                      with pH
       B **True**      predominantly pharmacodynamic interaction
       C **True**      aspirin is acetylsalicylic acid which is first
                      metabolised to salicylic acid
       D **True**      at lower doses is hyperuricaemic
       E **False**     powerful antipyretic unlike paracetamol

9.11  A **True**      mechanism not clear
       B **False**     allopurinol reduces the clearance of both 6MP and
                      azathioprine and may thus produce toxic effects
       C **False**     combined therapy may be necessary in some
                      patients
       D **True**      allopurinol will always reduce serum urate, whether
                      it is due to chemotherapy or starvation or other
                      causes
       E **False**     the prevalence of rashes particularly is higher in such
                      renal failure patients

9.12  A **True**      suspension given frequently is indicated
       B **True**      cream with or without pessaries, tablets and
                      treatment for partner
       C **False**     nystatin is too toxic to be given systemically.
                      Amphotericin B given i.v., although toxic, should be
                      used
       D **False**     oral amphotericin B should be used. This is absorbed
                      and acts systemically
       E **False**     systemic treatment needed

9.13  A **False**     no evidence that this dose will affect blood pressure
       B **False**     steroids will, however, suppress the inflammation of
                      acute gout
       C **True**      antituberculous therapy would be required if
                      treatment is to be prolonged
       D **True**      although the role of steroids in the pathogenesis of
                      peptic ulcer is uncertain delayed healing is likely
       E **True**      dissemination is a risk (producing satellite lesions or
                      full-blown chicken pox)

9.14  A **True**      direct action on smooth muscle
       B **False**     therapeutic effect is due to analgesic effect. Also has
                      an antidiuretic effect, reducing ureteric peristalsis
                      and thus smooth muscle spasm
       C **True**      shorter duration of action and reduced potency
                      probable explanation
       D **True**      as for C
       E **False**     two-hourly administration may be necessary because
                      of the short half-life

**9.15  The following drugs may produce unwanted effects on the fetus when given in the third trimester of pregnancy**

  A  carbimazole
  B  folic acid
  C  ferrous gluconate
  D  ampicillin
  E  tetracyclines

**9.16  Phenytoin**

  A  is preferred to phenobarbitone in both generalised and temporal lobe epilepsy
  B  may cause gingival hypertrophy
  C  may cause ataxia
  D  is superior to ethosuximide in the treatment of petit mal epilepsy
  E  may cause hirsutism

**9.17  When prescribing phenytoin**

  A  there is a narrow therapeutic index
  B  dosage should be gradually increased by total daily dose increments of 100 mg
  C  a loading dose may be given intravenously or orally
  D  the time taken to halve the serum concentration is independent of dose
  E  once daily dosing is usually inadequate

**9.18  Tricyclic antidepressants**

  A  often produce dryness of the mouth
  B  often produce sleeplessness
  C  cause profound coma with small pupils when taken in overdosage
  D  block monoamine uptake at adrenergic nerve terminals
  E  antagonise the antihypertensive effect of adrenergic receptor blockers

**9.19  A collagen disease syndrome (e.g. systemic lupus erythematosus) can be caused by**

  A  hyaluronidase
  B  procaineamide
  C  hydralazine
  D  prazosin
  E  pheytoin

9.15  A **True**      fetal hypothyroidism
       B **False**     may be beneficial in protecting against neural tube
                      defects
       C **False**     any ferrous salt may be used
       D **False**     probably the broad-spectrum antibiotic of choice in
                      pregnancy
       E **True**      deposited in bones and teeth — the latter producing
                      cosmetic disfigurement

9.16  A **True**      phenobarbitone is no longer a drug of first choice for
                      any indication
       B **True**      this adverse effect seems only to be a problem when
                      gingivitis is chronically present
       C **True**      dose-related effect. Common manifestation of
                      therapeutic intoxication
       D **False**     ethosuximide is the drug of choice
       E **True**      usually seen with chronic therapy over several years

9.17  A **True**
       B **False**     once doses exceed 200–300 mg daily, increments
                      should be only 50 mg
       C **True**      doses of 1 gram or more may be needed to obtain
                      therapeutic concentrations on starting therapy by
                      either route
       D **False**     non-linear (dose-dependent) kinetics is seen in some
                      patients even within the therapeutic range. In the
                      toxic range it may take a week to halve the serum
                      concentration
       E **False**     even when kinetics are linear, the half-life is long
                      enough to justify once daily dosing

9.18  A **True**      dose-related effect
       B **False**     drowsiness is caused by most of these drugs
       C **False**     the anticholinergic action produces large pupils in
                      such patients
       D **True**
       E **False**     tricyclics block uptake of adrenergic neurone blockers
                      (and thus antagonise their effect). Receptor blockers
                      act directly

9.19  A **False**
       B **True**      rarely used in UK now
       C **True**      fast acetylators virtually never develop this
                      complication
       D **False**
       E **True**

**9.20    The following classes of drugs are among the more common causes of photosensitivity**

A    tetracyclines
B    non-steroidal anti-inflammatories
C    beta-blockers
D    alpha-blockers
E    sulphonamides

9.20 A **True**

B **True**    for some agents (e.g. benoxaprofen, now withdrawn)
nearly 1 in 2 patients were affected in some way

C **False**

D **False**

E **True**    this is one of the reasons that trimethoprim alone is
favoured in urinary tract infections versus
cotrimoxazole (trimethoprim plus
sulphamethoxazole, a sulphonamide)

# Chapter 10

**10.1** During treatment for Hodgkin's disease, a 32 year old man is prescribed allopurinol for prevention of gout. The following statements are true

A gout may be precipitated

B by inhibiting xanthine oxidase, it decreases the production of hypoxanthine

C a dose-related skin rash may occur

D the concurrent use of probenecid may decrease the dose of allopurinol required

E frusemide will antagonise the effects of allopurinol

**10.2** The following statements relating to pharmacokinetic terms are true

A elimination half-life ($T$): for most drugs, the amount eliminated from the plasma is directly proportional to the amount present

B bioavailability: this describes the amount of drug which is absorbed following administration

C the volume of distribution ($V_d$): is inversely proportional to the clearance of a drug

D clearance: is calculated by dividing the dose administered by the area under the time concentration curve

E first order kinetics: the elimination half-life (T[) of a drug is independent of the dose

**10.3** The following statements are true

A the excretion of phenobarbitone is not altered in the presence of renal impairment

B barbiturates are mainly metabolised by microsomal liver enzymes

C tolerance may develop to barbiturates on repeated administration

D chlormethiazole may be useful in the management of acute withdrawal from barbiturates

E amylobarbitone increases the proportion of rapid eye movement sleep (REM)

10.1  A **True**   a drug-induced exacerbation of this condition may
                   also be seen with probenecid
      B **False**  by inhibiting xanthine oxidase, it decreases the
                   production of xanthine and uric acid
      C **True**
      D **True**   probenecid inhibits the reabsorption of uric acid by
                   the renal tubules
      E **True**   frusemide may cause hyperuricaemia but this effect
                   appears to be more common with thiazide diuretics

10.2  A **True**
      B **False**  biovailability is the percentage of drug released from
                   a formulation that becomes available for biological
                   effect
      C **False**  volume of distribution ($V_d$) is directly proportional to
                   clearance of a drug
      D **True**
      E **True**

10.3  A **False**  up to 30% of phenobarbitone is excreted by the
                   kidneys
      B **True**
      C **True**   this reflects a more rapid metabolism and shorter
                   half-life due to induction of microsomal liver
                   enzymes
      D **True**   chlormethiazole has sedative and anticonvulsant
                   properties which are useful in the treatment of acute
                   withdrawal from alcohol, narcotic analgesics and
                   barbiturates
      E **False**  REM sleep is suppressed

**10.4    In a patient with a recent myocardial infarction**
    **A**   lignocaine should be prescribed immediately to prevent arrhythmias
    **B**   beta-adrenergic blockers cause a reduction in the recurrence rate of myocardial infarction
    **C**   warfarin may cause pericarditis
    **D**   amiodarone is now the treatment of choice for supraventricular tachycardia
    **E**   nifedipine may precipitate heart failure

**10.5    Overdose of iron may be associated with the following**
    **A**   hepatic necrosis
    **B**   shock
    **C**   marked gut upset
    **D**   48 hour delay in onset of symptoms
    **E**   parkinsonism

**10.6    Lithium**
    **A**   is used to treat severe anxiety
    **B**   may cause hypothyroidism
    **C**   may be associated with hyperthyroidism
    **D**   can cause renal damage given long term
    **E**   may cause blurred vision in overdose

**10.7    Amphetamine**
    **A**   when given orally raises both systolic and diastolic blood pressures
    **B**   prolongs duration of rapid eye movement (REM) sleep
    **C**   causes pupillary constriction
    **D**   improves physical performance in athletes
    **E**   treatment of acute amphetamine intoxication includes alkalinisation of the urine to facilitate excretion of the drug

10.4   A **False**   liognocaine has a negative inotropic effect which
                     could impair cardiac performance. It is used to treat
                     ventricular arrhythmias following myocardial
                     infarction
       B **True**
       C **False**   a pericardial effusion (containing blood) is a more
                     likely event when warfarin is taken
       D **False**   amiodarone is useful in the treatment of atrial
                     fibrillation associated with the Wolff-Parkinson-White
                     syndrome and in the long-term treatment of patients
                     with recurrent ventricular arrhythmias
       E **False**   nifedipine has negative inotropic effects but these are
                     unlikely to be significant when therapeutic doses are
                     used. In fact, a modest improvement in cardiac
                     output may be an accompaniment of treatment with
                     this drug

10.5   A **True**
       B **True**
       C **True**    a hypokalaemic alkalosis may develop secondary to
                     vomiting
       D **False**   signs and symptoms of iron poisoning usually
                     appear within a few hours after ingestion
       E **False**   manganese mining however may cause
                     parkinsonism

10.6   A **False**   lithium is used in the treatment of recurrent
                     depression and acute mania
       B **True**    a goitre and hypothyroidism may develop secondary
                     to an inhibitory effect on thyroid hormone synthesis
       C **True**    hyperthyroidism has been reported in patients on
                     lithium but this may not be a causal relationship
       D **True**
       E **True**    may also be associated with mental confusion,
                     dysarthria, seizures and focal neurological signs

10.7   A **True**
       B **False**   amphetamine delays the onset of REM sleep and is
                     useful in the treatment of narcolepsy which is
                     associated with an immediate onset of REM sleep
       C **False**   pupillary dilatation occurs
       D **True**    this improvement may be reversed by overdosage or
                     repeated usage of amphetamine
       E **False**   acidification of the urine increases the degree of
                     ionisation of amphetamine which is a weak base,
                     thereby decreasing the amount reabsorbed by the
                     renal tubule

**10.8    The following statements are true in relation to the excretion of drugs**

  A    inhalational anaesthetics are excreted mainly by the lungs
  B    because of good penetration into bile, sulphonamides are useful in biliary tract disease
  C    the kidney and gastrointestinal tract are the major routes of drug elimination
  D    during metabolism of the drug, an increase in lipid solubility will facilitate excretion
  E    alkalinisation of the urine hastens the renal excretion of phenobarbitone

**10.9    Angiotensin converting enzyme (ACE) inhibitors may cause the following effects**

  A    marked postural hypotension
  B    an increase in the level of aldosterone
  C    proteinuria
  D    leucopenia
  E    arterial vasodilatation

**10.10   The following drugs may interfere with the laboratory test for blood grouping**

  A    spironolactone
  B    dextran 70
  C    alpha-methyldopa
  D    mefanamic acid
  E    chlorpromazine

**10.11   Pupils may be dilated for ophthalmoscopy by the following drugs instilled into the conjunctival sac**

  A    cyclopentolate
  B    hypromellose
  C    acetazolamide
  D    homatropine
  E    pilocarpine

10.8  A  **True**   however, up to 15% of halothane may be
                    metabolised by the liver and excreted eventually by
                    the kidneys. Minor amounts of the drugs may be
                    excreted through the skin and mucous membranes
       B  **False**  sulphonamides readily enter pleural, peritoneal,
                    synovial and other body fluids, but penetration into
                    bile is poor
       C  **True**
       D  **False**  metabolism usually produces polar (water-soluble)
                    metabolites which facilitates excretion by the kidneys
                    and gut
       E  **True**   phenobarbitone, which is a weak acid, is ionised to a
                    greater extent when the urine has an alkaline pH.
                    This hastens excretion by the consequent decrease in
                    lipid solubility

10.9  A  **False**  as baroreceptor function and cardiovascular reflexes
                    are relatively unimpaired, postural hypotension does
                    not usually occur
       B  **False**  secretion of aldosterone is reduced but some output
                    of the hormone is maintained by other stimulating
                    factors such as ACTH
       C  **True**   more likely when patients have a history of renal
                    disease
       D  **True**   risk increased in renal disease or autoimmune
                    disorders such as SLE
       E  **True**

10.10 A  **False**  estimation of plasma cortisol by a fluorescent
                    method, and of digoxin by radioimmunoassay, may
                    be interfered with by spironolactone
       D  **True**   dextran facilitates red cell rouleaux formation and
                    therefore interferes with accurate cross-matching
       C  **True**   a positive Coomb's test with production of IgG may
                    occur
       D  **True**   an autoimmune haemolyte anaemia due to the
                    production of an antibody may occur
       E  **False**

10.11 A  **True**   by virtue of its antimuscarinic action
       B  **False**  hypromellose eye drops are employed as 'artificial
                    tears' for the treatment of chronic dry eyes such as in
                    Sjögren's syndrome
       C  **False**  acetazolamide reduces the production of aqueous
                    humour by inhibiting carbonic anhydrase. It is used
                    to lower intraocular pressure in glaucoma
       D  **True**   also interferes with accommodation
       E  **False**  causes pupillary constriction by virtue of its
                    muscarinic properties

**10.12  The following drug combinations should be avoided**

A   aspirin and warfarin
B   monoamine oxidase inhibitor (MAOI) and propranolol
C   captopril and frusemide
D   lithium and bendrofluazide
E   chlorpropamide and metformin

**10.13  During cardiopulmonary resuscitation, the following conditions may respond to the treatment indicated**

A   asystole — adrenaline
B   coarse ventricular fibrillation — lignocaine
C   ventricular tachycardia with no pulse — adrenaline
D   complete heart block — defibrillation
E   electromechanical dissociation — calcium chloride

**10.14  The oral contraceptive pill (combined preparation) may cause the following adverse effects**

A   impaired glucose tolerance
B   liver tumours
C   increased incidence of ovarian carcinoma
D   increase in the incidence of benign breast disease
E   hypertension

**10.15  Hypoglycaemia is a recognised complication during treatment with the following**

A   glucagon
B   diazoxide
C   tolbutamide
D   metformin
E   propranolol

10.12  A  **True**    aspirin may increase the risk of bleeding by several
                      mechanisms:
                      1. gastric irritation
                      2. reduction in platelet adhesion and aggregation
                      3. displacement of warfarin from its binding sites on
                         plasma proteins
       B  **True**    propranolol administration may be associated with
                      depression in some patients
       C  **False**   frusemide in doses up to 120 mg daily by mouth has
                      been shown to improve the antihypertensive effect of
                      captopril
       D  **True**    by reducing renal excretion of lithium, thiazides may
                      predispose patients to developing lithium toxicity
       E  **False**   combination therapy with a sulphonylurea and
                      metformin may be useful in the treatment of non-
                      insulin-dependent diabetes mellitus

10.13  A  **True**
       B  **True**
       C  **False**   the primary treatment in this case would be
                      lignocaine with direct current defribillation
       D  **False**   temporary electrical pacing would be a more
                      appropriate treatment. Use of isoprenaline is also of
                      benefit in some cases
       E  **True**    adrenaline and isoprenaline are also of use in this
                      condition

10.14  A  **True**
       B  **True**    the development of benign vascular adenomas is a
                      rare adverse effect of the 'pill', but usually these
                      regress on cessation of the drug
       C  **False**   an increased incidence of endometrial carcinoma in
                      premenopausal women has been reported
       D  **False**   there is a decreased incidence of benign breast
                      disease
       E  **True**    about 5% of women on the 'pill' develop
                      hypertension which usually resolves on stopping the
                      drug

10.15  A  **False**   glucagon causes an increase in the level of plasma
                      glucose
       B  **False**   causes hyperglycaemia
       C  **True**    tolbutamide is a first generation sulphonylurea urea
                      in the treatment of non-insulin-dependent diabetes
                      mellitus
       D  **False**   metformin, in therapeutic doses, has a glucose-
                      lowering effect in diabetes but does not cause
                      hypoglycaemia
       E  **False**   propranolol and other beta-antagonists delay/inhibit
                      recovery from hypoglycaemia, they do not cause it

**10.16  Chloroquine**
  A   usually has a therapeutic effect by two weeks of treatment in rheumatoid arthritis
  B   may cause deafness
  C   should not be given to patients over 55 years of age
  D   is useful in the treatment of systemic lupus erythematosis (SLE)
  E   should be given with quinine in severe malarial infection

**10.17  Excessive hair growth (hirsuties) may be associated with use of the following**
  A   carbimazole
  B   corticosteroids
  C   minoxidil
  D   heparin
  E   phenytoin

**10.18  In a 50-year-old diabetic prescribed metformin**
  A   nausea in the first two weeks of treatment may be troublesome
  B   alcohol is contraindicated
  C   an increase in weight is likely
  D   renal impairment is not a contraindication to treatment
  E   unsatisfactory blood sugar control warrants substituting metformin with phenformin

**10.19  The following drugs have been shown to be of use prophylactically in migraine**
  A   clonidine
  B   methysergide
  C   reserpine
  D   ergotamine
  E   propranolol

10.16 A **False**    subjective benefit from chloroquine begins at about 6
                     weeks of treatment, but objective improvement is not
                     seen until about 3 months after the start of treatment
      B **True**     permanent nerve deafness in adults has followed
                     high-dose chloroquine therapy. A more common
                     adverse effect is irreversible retinal damage
      C **True**     there is an increased risk of toxicity in the elderly
      D **True**     has a steroid-sparing effect in arthritis and skin
                     involvement due to SLE
      E **False**    in severe malarial infections (mainly due to
                     *Plasmodium falciparum*) chloroquine resistance is
                     likely and the primary treatment is with quinine given
                     by intravenous infusion

10.17 A **False**    causes hair loss (alopecia)
      B **True**     there is less convincing evidence that hirsuties
                     follows use of topical corticosteroid preparations
      C **True**     minoxidil may prove useful in the treatment of
                     certain forms of alopecia
      D **False**    causes alopecia
      E **True**

10.18 A **True**     the gastrointestinal side-effects of metformin may be
                     lessened if smaller doses of the drug are taken
                     initially and if the drug is taken with food
      B **True**     alcohol potentiates the action of metformin and may
                     give rise to dangerous hypoglycaemia
      C **False**    metformin has an anorectic effect. Sulphonylurea
                     treatment often leads to an increase in weight in
                     patients
      D **False**    metformin is excreted virtually unchanged in the
                     urine. Renal impairment would predispose a patient
                     to developing lactic acidosis
      E **False**    phenformin has been withdrawn from the UK market
                     because of its association with lactic acidosis in
                     patients receiving it. Metformin, in therapeutic doses,
                     when given to patients with normal hepatic and renal
                     function is said to be associated with a much smaller
                     risk of developing this serious and often fatal side
                     effect

10.19 A **True**
      B **True**     methysergide is, however, not useful for the
                     treatment of acute attacks
      C **False**    has no place in the treatment of migraine
      D **False**    only useful in the treatment of acute attacks
      E **True**     atenolol and nadolol appear to be effective from the
                     prophylactic point of view as well

**10.20  The following statements about the use of drugs in the elderly are true**

   **A**   adverse drugs reactions are less common

   **B**   an increased risk of bleeding is present during warfarin treatment

   **C**   nitrazepan given in doses used for the young may produce prolonged daytime confusion

   **D**   the use of chlorpropamide should be avoided

   **E**   there is little evidence for any major changes in drug absorption from the gastrointestinal tract

10.20 A **False**   more common
      B **True**    elderly patients when compared to the young are
                    also more likely to bleed during heparin treatment
      C **True**    because of its relatively long half-life of 18–29 h and
                    the increased sensitivity of elderly patients to
                    benzodiazepines, prolonged effects may be seen
      D **True**    chlorpropamide has a half-life of about 33–36 h and
                    duration of action up to 60 h. This predisposes
                    elderly patients especially to unwanted
                    hypoglycaemia
      E **True**

# Chapter 11

**11.1 Cyclosporin A**

  **A** acts specifically on B lymphocytes
  **B** can only be given intravenously
  **C** may be given prophylactically to reduce rejection of organ transplants
  **D** causes little bone marrow suppression
  **E** should be avoided in severe renal impairment

**11.2 A 40-year-old patient in cardiogenic shock is given an intravenous infusion of dopamine. The following statements are true**

  **A** an increase in glomerular filtration rate (GFR) may occur
  **B** in high doses dopamine may cause renal vasoconstriction
  **C** the infusion bottle should be protected from light during administration
  **D** excessive tachycardia may require the administration of propranolol
  **E** prolonged use of dopamine may cause gangrene of the fingers

**11.3 Vitamin C (ascorbic acid)**

  **A** is used in the treatment of sulphaemoglobinaemia
  **B** when taken in large doses can cause hyperparathyroidism
  **C** deficiency may cause a macrocytic anaemia
  **D** catalyses the conversion of hydroxproline to proline during collagen synthesis
  **E** is measured using intracellular erythrocyte concentrations

11.1  A **False**   cyclosporin A is thought to act by blocking an early
                    stage in the activation of cytotoxic T lymphocytes. It
                    also inhibits the production of interferon by
                    lymphocytes
      B **False**   may also be given via the oral route as a solution
      C **True**    has also been used with some success in bone
                    marrow transplantation
      D **True**    unlike other immunosuppressants
      E **True**    renal function becomes impaired or may worsen
                    during treatment with cyclosporin A

11.2  A **True**    administration of low doses of dopamine causes an
                    increase in GFR, sodium excretion, and renal blood
                    flow
      B **True**    this is due to stimulation of alpha (?) receptors in the
                    renal vasculature
      C **False**   this precaution usually is applied to the
                    administration of sodium nitroprusside to prevent
                    degradation yielding cyanide
      D **False**   because of dopamine's short half-life (about 2 min)
                    any unwanted effects usually disappear when the
                    infusion is slowed or stopped. Propranolol, because
                    it inhibits sympathetic stimulation of the heart (by
                    beta$_1$ blockade) may actually worsen the situation
      E **True**    due to chronic alpha (?) stimulation of digital vessels
                    leading to intense vasoconstriction

11.3  A **False**   because of its reducing properties ascorbic acid is
                    useful in the treatment of methaemoglobinaemia
      B **False**
      C **True**    due to a block in the conversion of folic acid to folinic
                    acid
      D **False**   during the synthesis of collagen ascorbic acid plays a
                    role in the hydroxylation of proline to hydroxyproline
      E **False**   levels of ascorbic acid in leucocytes are taken to
                    indicate whether there is an adequate supply of the
                    vitamin

**11.4**    **A 34-year-old man is admitted for a hernia repair. He is given suxamethonium during induction of anaesthesia. The following statements are true:**

    **A**    suxamethonium is a non-depolarising neuromuscular blocker

    **B**    the action of suxamethonium may be reversed by neostigmine

    **C**    prolonged paralysis may occur

    **D**    if halothane is also used, a dangerous rise in temperature may occur

    **E**    because of the nicotinic actions of suxamethonium, atropine is usually given before its use

**11.5**    **Carbenoxolone**

    **A**    is ineffective in healing gastric ulcers

    **B**    causes hypokalaemia

    **C**    has an enhanced therapeutic action when taken with antacids

    **D**    inhibits gastric acid production

    **E**    aggravates the treatment of hypertension

**11.6**    **Amiodarone**

    **A**    is a class 1 antiarrhythmic agent according to the Vaughn-Williams classification

    **B**    has no place in the treatment of ventricular arrhythmias

    **C**    is useful in the treatment of the Wolff-Parkinson-White (WPW) syndrome

    **D**    may be associated with the development of corneal deposits

    **E**    may interfere with the interpretation of thyroid function tests

11.4  A **False**   causes muscular paralysis by depolarisation at the
                     neuromuscular junction
      B **False**   neostigmine reverses the action of curare but may
                     prolong the depolarisation caused by
                     suxamethonium, by inhibiting acetylcholinesterase
      C **True**    in about 1 in 2800 of the population
                     pseudocholinesterase, an enzyme responsible for the
                     metabolism of suxamethonium, has poor activity
                     which results in prolonged apnoea
      D **True**    this condition is called malignant hyperpyrexia which
                     has a familial tendency. Other drugs implicated in
                     this condition are cyclopropane, chloroform and
                     diethyl ether
      E **False**   suxamethonium exhibits muscarinic actions which
                     require the use of atropine beforehand

11.5  A **False**   carbenoxolone was the first drug to have a healing
                     effect on gastric ulcers. It is less effective in healing
                     duodenal ulcers
      B **True**    due to its mineralocorticoid activity
      C **False**   carbenoxolone is a weak acid and is mainly
                     unionised and therefore highly lipid soluble in the
                     acid pH of the stomach. An increase in pH caused by
                     taking an antacid would consequently impair
                     absorption of the drug
      D **False**   carbenoxolone exerts its therapeutic effects by
                     altering the mucosal barrier to acid, suppressing the
                     activation of pepsinogen, and by a possible effect on
                     certain gastroprotective prostaglandins
      E **True**    along with hypokalaemia, other mineral corticoid
                     effects include fluid retention and hypertension

11.6  A **False**   amiodarone is a class III agent and exerts its
                     therapeutic action by prolonging the duration of the
                     action potential and the effective refractory period in
                     the atria and ventricles
      B **False**   amiodarone is useful in the long-term treatment of
                     patients with recurrent ventricular arrhythmias
      C **True**    this is a specific indication especially when atrial
                     fibrillation is associated with the WPW syndrome
      D **True**    asymptomatic corneal microdeposits develop in
                     most patients receiving amiodarone. They are
                     usually reversible on stopping the drug
      E **True**    amiodarone contains iodine which may interfere with
                     the metabolic conversion of the thyroid hormones
                     both hypo- and hyperthyroidism have been reported

**11.7    Treatment of the following conditions may predispose the patient to developing proteinuria**

A   hypertension
B   peptic ulcer
C   diabetes mellitus
D   Wilson's disease
E   rheumatoid arthritis

**11.8    The following drugs cause visual loss by damage to the retina**

A   tetracycline
B   digoxin
C   ethambutol
D   chloroquine
E   atropine

**11.9    Morphine**

A   causes pupillary constriction
B   produces nausea by a direct irritant effect on the gastric mucosa
C   undergoes significant first-pass metabolism
D   is useful as an analgesic in acute pancreatitis
E   should be avoided in asthma

11.7  A **True**    hydralazine and β-adrenoceptor blockers may
                    predispose the patient to developing drug-induced
                    systemic lupus nephritis with consequent
                    proteinuria. Thiazides and frusemide have been
                    implicated in some cases of nephrotic syndrome.
                    Captopril may cause proteinuria

      B **False**

      C **False**   of course, patients may develop proteinuria as a
                    result of the progression of diabetes

      D **True**    penicillamine which increases the urinary excretion
                    of copper in Wilson's disease may cause renal
                    damage and resulting proteinuria

      E **True**    both gold and penicillamine, which is also used in
                    rheumatoid arthritis, may cause renal damage
                    leading to proteinuria. Pain-killers, such as aspirin,
                    may cause a nephropathy (analgesic nephropathy)

11.8  A **False**   tetracyclines have, however, been implicated in
                    producing papilloedema

      B **True**    cardiac glycosides are known to cause irreversible
                    pigmentary changes in the retina associated with
                    visual loss. Changes in colour vision may also occur

      C **False**   ethambutol is associated with causing visual loss due
                    to optic neuropathy rather than retinal damage

      D **True**    visual loss by retinal and macular(?) pigmentation
                    occurs. Patients on chloroquine should have regular
                    fundal examinations carried out

      E **False**   however, atropine has been associated with diplopia,
                    mydriasis and dry eyes in patients receiving the drug

11.9  A **True**    the exact mechanism is unknown but may be due to
                    a stimulatory effect on the Edinger-Westphal nucleus
                    which supplies parasympathetic nerve fibres to the
                    pupil

      B **False**   nausea and vomiting after morphine are due to a
                    direct stimulation of the chemoreceptor trigger zone
                    in the medulla

      C **True**    because of hepatic metabolism, the bioavailability of
                    the drug is considerably less after administration by
                    the oral route than when given intravenously.
                    Conjugation with glucuronic acid is the major
                    metabolic pathway

      D **False**   morphine causes an increase in pressure of the
                    biliary tree and may give rise to further epigastric
                    pain due to biliary colic

      E **True**    morphine causes a depression of the respiratory
                    centre and cough reflex and may release histamine.
                    All these may have deleterious effects in asthma

**11.10    In ethylene glycol poisoning**
  A    the initial clinical picture resembles acute ethanol intoxication
  B    a metabolic alkalosis occurs
  C    hypocalcaemia may develop
  D    gastric aspiration and lavage is contraindicated
  E    ethanol should be given

**11.11    The following drugs are contraindicated in asthma**
  A    verapamil
  B    atenolol
  C    diazepam
  D    sodium cromoglycate
  E    aspirin

**11.12    Somatostatin**
  A    is secreted by the pituitary gland
  B    lowers growth hormone levels in acromegaly
  C    may have a use in the treatment of bleeding from oesophageal varices
  D    promotes insulin secretion
  E    has been implicated in causing dementia by being contaminated with slow viruses

11.10 A **True**   there is nausea, vomiting, haematemesis, convulsions and coma. Pulmonary oedema and acute renal failure may develop

     B **False**   metabolism of ethylene glycol yields formic acid giving rise to a metabolic acidosis

     C **True**   this may be associated with the formation of calcium oxalate crystals and give rise to tetany

     D **False**   this is a useful measure in the early stages following ingestion of the drug

     E **True**   ethanol competes for the same metabolic pathway as ethylene glycol. It is usually given orally followed by an intravenous infusion

11.11 A **False**

     B **True**   although atenolol is considered to be a cardioselective $\beta_1$ adrenergic blocker, bronchospasm by blockade of bronchial $\beta_2$ receptors may still occur

     C **True**   respiratory depression is a potential adverse effect of treatment with diazepam and is obviously more dangerous in chronic lung disease and asthma

     D **False**   sodium cromoglycate acts on the mast cell to prevent release of histamine, leucotrienes and other agents which cause bronchoconstriction

     E **True**   up to about 2% of asthmatics appear to be sensitive to aspirin and other drugs such as indomethacin and may develop symptoms of wheezing associated with urticaria and rhinorrhoea

11.12 A **False**   somatostatin is a tetradecapeptide which is secreted by the hypothalamus but other areas such as the spinal cord and pancreas have been shown to contain the hormone

     B **True**   growth hormone secretion is inhibited (as well as TSH and ACTH)

     C **True**   somatostatin has been shown to raise gastric pH to 7–7.5 and reduce splanchnic blood flow. It has compared favourably with cimetidine in controlling haemorrhage from bleeding peptic ulcers

     D **False**   inhibits secretion of insulin

     E **False**   a number of cases of dementia due to Jakob-Creutzfeldt disease have been reported following growth hormone replacement therapy. Human growth hormone produced by bacterial recombinant DNA techniques is now available

**11.13** **A syndrome resembling systemic lupus erythematosis (SLE) has been reported following use of:**

A   chlorpromazine
B   phenytoin
C   cimetidine
D   digoxin
E   hydralazine

**11.14** **The following infections are likely to responde to the antibiotic indicated**

A   Legionnaires' disease — erythromycin
B   meningococcal meningitis — penicillin G
C   gonorrhoea — amoxycillin
D   aspergillosis — griseofulvin
E   leptospirosis — cotrimoxazole

**11.15** **Patients on warfarin are at increased risk from bleeding when the following drugs are also taken**

A   rifampicin
B   oral contraceptive pill
C   phenylbutazone
D   aspirin
E   cimetidine

11.13 A **True**
      B **True**
      C **False**
      D **False**
      E **True**     drug-induced SLE tends to be less severe than spontaneous SLE and may be reversible after the drug has been withdrawn. However, contrary to previous reports, renal involvement may occur and in some cases be severe

11.14 A **True**     rifampicin may also be effective as an additional drug in this condition
      B **True**     chloramphenicol is an alternative antibiotic
      C **True**     procaine penicillin (i.m.), tetracyclines or ampicillin are alternatives
      D **False**    griseofulvin has no activity on the *Aspergillus* species
      E **False**    for a number of reasons, there appears to be a great lack of convincing evidence for any particular antibiotic in leptospirosis. However, most clinicians would advise treatment with parenteral penicillin or tetracycline

11.15 A **False**    in the presence of rifampicin, warfarin has a reduced anticoagulant effect because of inhibition of its hepatic metabolism
      B **False**    oral contraceptives increase plasma levels of factor VII and can reduce the anticoagulant effect of warfarin
      C **True**     phenylbutazone inhibits the hepatic metabolism of warfarin thereby potentiating its action. Other effects such as displacement of warfarin from protein binding sites, impaired platelet aggregation and development of peptic ulceration also increase the risk of haemorrhage
      D **True**     aspirin may enhance the anticoagulant effect of warfarin by a number of mechanisms similar to those of phenylbutazone: displacement of warfarin from protein binding sites, antiplatelet effects, increase risk of peptic ulceration
      E **True**     cimetidine, although useful in the management of upper gastrointestinal haemorrhage secondary to peptic ulceration, may inhibit the hepatic metabolism of warfarin and therefore potentiate its action

**11.16**   A 27-year-old woman was admitted with a 10-day history of diarrhoea. Rectal biopsy showed features of pseudomembranous colitis. Previous treatment with the following antibiotics may have been responsible

  A   metronidazole
  B   lincomycin
  C   vancomycin
  D   clindamycin
  E   ampicillin

**11.17**   A patient with a phaeochromocytoma should not be given the following

  A   morphine
  B   a thiazide diuretic
  C   nitrazepam
  D   phenoxybenzamine
  E   phenelzine

**11.18**   Drugs which should be avoided in patients with liver failure include

  A   aspirin
  B   chlorpromazine
  C   chlormethiazole
  D   neomycin
  E   metformin

11.16 A **False**
      B **True**
      C **False**    vancomycin is usually the treatment of choice.
                     Metronidaxole, bacitracin and cholestyramine may
                     also be used with some benefit
      D **True**
      E **True**     this condition is caused by a toxin released from
                     strains of a bacteriuum, *Clostridium difficile*. The
                     colitis does not appear to be dose-related and may
                     occur after parenteral or oral treatment with
                     antibiotics

11.17 A **True**     this was a difficult question. Morphine may release
                     noradrenaline from neurones and cause a dangerous
                     increase in blood pressure in a patient with a
                     phaeochromocytoma
      B **False**
      C **False**
      D **False**    because of its alpha-blocking properties,
                     phenoxybenzamine has been used in the treatment
                     of hypertension due to phaeochromocytomas
      E **True**     phenelzine is a monoamine oxidase inhibitor. When
                     patients on this drug take tyramine-containing foods,
                     a dangerous increase in blood pressure may occur
                     due to excessive catecholamine release. Phenelzine,
                     by preventing breakdown of catecholamines, would
                     worsen the hypertension in phaeochromocytomas

11.18 A **True**     aspirin has antiplatelet actions which increase the
                     risk of haemorrhage. Also, there is evidence for a
                     direct, dose-dependent, hepatotoxic effect of aspirin
      B **True**     chlorpromazine is known to cause cholestatic
                     jaundice which may be prolonged up to three
                     months in some cases. It is also implicated in causing
                     a dose-dependent injury to the liver. Apart from
                     these, chlorpromazine and other phenothiazins may
                     precipitate hepatic encephalopathy in patients with
                     liver failure
      C **False**    chlormethiazole may be useful as a sedative to
                     control withdrawal symptoms in patients with
                     alcoholic liver failure. It must, however, be given in
                     reduced doses
      D **False**    neomycin has proved effective in lowering
                     gastrointestinal ammonia formation by its action on
                     the bacterial flora and is used in the treatment of
                     hepatic coma
      E **True**     there is an increased risk of lactic acidosis

**11.19  Gold**

    **A**  is usually given orally
    **B**  is prescribed on a once-daily basis
    **C**  causes skin rashes in up to 15% of patients
    **D**  may cause proteinuria
    **E**  arrests the progress of the disease in rheumatoid arthritis

**11.20  A 39-year-old man is admitted into hospital because of urinary retention. Previous treatment with the following could have been responsible**

    **A**  amitriptyline
    **B**  methyldopa
    **C**  disopyramide
    **D**  cimetidine
    **E**  captopril

11.19 A **False**    absorption by the oral route is erratic and
                     unpredictable. It is given by intramuscular injection
      B **False**    gold has a long half-life and accumulates with
                     repeated administration. It is given weekly for one
                     month, and then given monthly until a maximum
                     total dose has been givén
      C **True**
      D **True**     during gold therapy, damage to the proximal
                     convoluted tubule may occur giving rise to
                     proteinuria. Membranous glomenlomephritis may
                     also occur
      E **True**     because of its toxicity, gold should not be used to
                     treat mild rheumatoid arthritis. Other drugs which
                     alter the progression of this disease include
                     penicillamine

11.20 A **True**     due to its anticholinergic action
      B **False**    methyldopa may interfere with sexual function by
                     causing failure of ejaculation
      C **True**     due to its anticholinergic action
      D **False**    causes gynaecomastia and hyperprolactinaemia
                     which may lead to impotence
      E **False**

# Chapter 12

**12.1   Impotence is a recognised complication of treatment with**

    **A**  prazosin
    **B**  bromocriptine
    **C**  methyldopa
    **D**  ranitidine
    **E**  chlorpromazine

**12.2   The following drugs are useful in the condition mentioned**

    **A**  calcitonin — Paget's disease of bone
    **B**  atenolol — Prinzmetal's angina
    **C**  streptokinase — major pulmonary embolism
    **D**  doxapram — status epilepticus
    **E**  penicillamime — chronic active hepatitis

**12.3   The following drugs are 'safe' in pregnancy**

    **A**  cotrimoxazole
    **B**  amiodarone
    **C**  penicillin
    **D**  indomethacin
    **E**  methyldopa

12.1    A **True**    by virtue of its alpha₁-adrenoceptor blocking action
        B **False**   bromocriptine (a dopamine receptor agonsit) is used in the treatment of impotence due to hyperprolactinaemia
        C **True**    other antihypertensive agents which can cause impotence include clonidine, bethanidine and guanethidine
        D **False**   cimetidine, another H₂-blocker, can cause hyperprolactinaemia but this has not been seen with ranitidine treatment
        E **True**    causes hyperprolactinaemia by dopamine blockade

12.2    A **True**    calcitonin reduced both alkaline phosphatase activity and urinary excretion of hydroxyproline in Paget's disease and thereby reduces bone resorption
        B **False**   in Prinzmetal's angina associated with coronary artery spasm, β-adrenergic blockade by atenolol can make the situation worse by allowing unopposed alpha-adrenergic coronary artery constriction to occur
        C **True**    streptokinase is a plasminogen activator and indirectly increases lysis of the fibrin clot seen in pulmonary embolism
        D **False**   doxapram may cause convulsions especially when given in high doses. It is used as a respiratory stimulant
        E **True**    corticosteroids and azathioprine are other drugs used in this condition

12.3    A **False**   may cause neonatal haemolysis and methaemoglobinaemia. There is also an increased risk of kernicterus in jaudiced neonates
        B **False**   may predispose to neonatal goitre
        C **True**
        D **False**   possible risk of pulmonary hypertension by inducing premature closure of the fetal ductus arteriosus. There may also be a delayed onset and increased duration of labour
        E **True**

**12.4    Chlorpropamide**
A    is associated with an alcohol-related flushing syndrome
B    has a short duration of action
C    should be given in reduced doses in pregnancy
D    may cause hyponatraemia
E    causes cholestatic jaundice

**12.5    A child is admitted into hospital having swallowed half a cupful of paraquat. The following statements are true:**
A    painful ulceration of the mouth and lips may appear 36–48 hours after ingestion
B    a suspension of Fuller's Earth is the single most useful treatment
C    plasma paraquat concentrations are not helpful in predicting outcome
D    renal failure is a well-recognised complication
E    oxygen treatment may be useful

**12.6    Prazosin**
A    may cause severe hypotension and collapse after the first dose
B    mainly acts by blocking presynaptic alpha$_1$-adrenergic neurones
C    acts on both the arterial and venous sides of the circulation
D    causes a marked reflex tachycardia
E    causes a marked rise in the level of plasma renin

12.4  A **True**    occurs in about 33% of patients taking
                    chlorpropamide. Autosomal dominant basis. Usually
                    only seen in patients with non-insulin-dependent
                    diabetes mellitus
      B **False**   the half-life is about 33–36 h and the duration of
                    action may be as long as 60 h
      C **False**   may cause neonatal hypoglycaemia
      D **True**    chlorpropamide stimulates antidiuretic hormone
                    (ADH) release which leads to dilutional
                    hyponatraemia and water intoxication in some cases
      E **True**    25% of patients on chlorpropamide develop
                    abnormal liver function tests but frank (?) jaundice is
                    estimated to occur in 0.5% of patients

12.5  A **True**
      B **True**    gastric aspiration and lavage followed by oral
                    administration of Fuller's Earth as a 30% suspension
                    is usually carried out initially. Further paraquat may
                    be removed by haemoperfusion or haemodialysis if
                    necessary
      C **False**   concentrations in the blood do appear to have
                    prognostic significance. Paraquat can be measure by
                    radioimmunoassay or gas chromatography
      D **True**
      E **False**   paraquat causes alveolar oedema, cellular infiltration
                    and progressive fibrosis of the lungs; oxygen therapy
                    tends to accentuate these effects

12.6  A **True**    this 'first dose' effect is characterised by hypotension
                    with loss of consciousness occurring 30–90 min after
                    the first dose in about 1% of patients taking an initial
                    dose of 2 mg
      B **False**   competitively blocks vascular postsynaptic $alpha_1$-
                    adrenergic receptors
      C **True**
      D **False**   at rest, prazosin reduces arterial pressure and
                    peripheral resistance, but produces little or no
                    tachycardia. A mild tachycardia can occur, however,
                    on standing
      E **False**   renin levels, unlike with hydralazine, are not raised
                    during prazosin treatment

**12.7    Prostacyclin**

A    is a potent vasoconstrictor
B    prevents platelet aggregation
C    works by elevating intracellular cyclic AMP
D    helps to protect the integrity of the stomach lining
E    is destroyed by phospholipase $A_2$

**12.8    Theophylline**

A    works by increasing the breakdown of cyclic AMP
B    has a positive inotropic effect
C    causes an increase in glomerular filtration rate (GFR)
D    needs to given at a reduced dose in renal impairment
E    when given intravenously, is useful in the management of acute asthma

**12.9    In the treatment of grand mal epilepsy**

A    in the first instance, prevention of further seizures should always be attempted using a single drug regimen
B    hypocalcaemia may develop following phenytoin administration
C    carbamazepine, unlike phenytoin, does not cause ataxia, diplopia and blurred vision during long-term administration
D    patients who develop liver disease may need a reduction in the dose of phenytoin to prevent toxicity
E    sodium valproate is ineffective

12.7  A **False**  causes vasodilatation
      B **True**   its effects on vascular smooth muscle and platelets
                   tend to be opposite to those of thromboxane $A_2$
      C **True**   an increase in intracellular cyclic AMP inhibits
                   platelet aggregation
      D **True**   prostacyclin has a number of effects on the stomach:
                   inhibits gastric acid secretion stimulated by feeding
                   or gastrin; increases mucus secretion; may have an
                   effect on altering blood flow to the stomach lining
      E **False**  phospholipase $A_2$ is a lysosomal enzyme which
                   hydrolyses phosphatidylcholine to lysolecithin and
                   fatty acids

12.8  A **False**  cyclic AMP levels are raised due to inhibition of
                   phosphodiesterase by theophylline
      B **True**   in therapeutic doses, theophylline produces a rise in
                   heart rate in normal subjects as well as an increase in
                   contractile force
      C **True**
      D **False**  the major route of elimination is by hepatic
                   metabolism
      E **True**   causes bronchodilatation

12.9  A **True**   the ideal antiepileptic regimen would involve using
                   one drug only which suppresses all seizures without
                   causing any unwanted side-effects
      B **True**   osteomalacia may also occur. This may be the result
                   of altered vitamin D metabolism and intestinal
                   absorption of calcium by phenytoin
      C **False**  other adverse effects include nausea, vomiting,
                   aplastic anaemia, hypersensitivity reactions and
                   retention of fluid is seen as a late complication of
                   treatment
      D **True**   phenytoin is extensively metabolised by the hepatic
                   microsomal enzyme system and any disturbance by
                   liver disease increases the risk of toxicity
      E **False**

**12.10   In the treatment of hypertension**

    **A**   hyperlipidaemia can occur within three weeks of treatment with thiazides

    **B**   bumetanide may cause deafness

    **C**   patients with low renin values are more responsive to beta-blockers

    **D**   guanethidine works by blocking the uptake of noradrenalin into the sympathetic nerve terminal

    **E**   methyldopa exerts its hypotensive effect mainly by an action on peripheral $alpha_1$ adrenergic neurons

**12.11   In designing a double-blind controlled clinical trial**

    **A**   the doctor knows what treatment each patient is taking

    **B**   a placebo must always be included in the design of the study even if the disease is serious

    **C**   the drug to be investigated must already have been given to normal volunteers

    **D**   if the results achieve no statistical significance, the drug studied has no therapeutic value

    **E**   all treatments used should be identical in appearance

**12.12   The following statements about ketoconazole are true**

    **A**   may be used in normal doses in patients with liver disease

    **B**   is effective in the treatment of candidiasis

    **C**   can be safely used in pregnancy

    **D**   it increases the rate of metabolism of rifampicin

    **E**   is an alternative to metronidazole in the treatment of giardiasis

12.10  A  **True**
    B  **True**    a transient form of deafness may occur (also seen following frusemide), but permanent deafness may occur during treatment with ethacrynic acid
    C  **False**   patients with high renin values are more sensitive to treatment with beta-adrenoceptor blockers. Patients with low renin values tend to be more sensitive to diuretic treatment
    D  **False**   guanethidine is an adrenergic neurone blocker which works by inhibiting noradrenaline release from presynaptic sympathetic nerve endings. During chronic treatment, nerve endings become depleted of noradrenaline as well
    E  **False**   the hypotensive effect of methyldopa is thought to originate in the central nervous system and be mainly due to its conversion to alphamethylnoradrenaline, a potent $alpha_2$ adrenergic agonist, thereby reducing sympathetic outflow from the brain

12.11  A  **False**   in a double-blind trial, neither patient, investigator nor the individual who evaluates the results is aware of which treatment the patient is receiving
    B  **False**   patients cannot be assigned on ethical grounds to only a placebo if there exists an alternative recognised therapy of established efficacy
    C  **False**   for the UK. In Sweden and the USA, however, properties of a new drug must first be investigated in normal subjects before the drug is given to patients. However, in practice most drugs are tried first in normals in the UK
    D  **False**   statistical tests assess the strength for a genuine difference in response to a particular treatment but cannot say whether a drug has a therapeutic effect or not
    E  **True**   if there is a difference then a placebo effect may be introduced, e.g. coloured tablets may evoke a better placebo response than white placebos

12.12  A  **False**   ketoconazole is directly hepatotoxic. Also, because it is metabolised by the liver, it may accumulate in liver disease
    B  **True**   other uses include treatment of dermatophyte and systemic fungal infections. It is not effective in infection due to aspergillus
    C  **False**   has potential serious toxicity
    D  **False**   by inducing hepatic microsomal enzymes, rifampicin increases the metabolic clearance of ketoconazole
    E  **False**   ketoconazole has no place in the treatment of infections due to *Giardia lamblia*

**12.13  The following side effects may be seen with insulin treatment**
A  lipohypertrophy
B  lipoatrophy
C  production of islet-cell antibodies
D  mental confusion
E  hypokalaemia

**12.14  The following drugs may cause hepatic cirrhosis**
A  glibenclamide
B  ranitidine
C  methyldopa
D  isoniazid
E  aspirin

**12.15  Trigeminal neuralgia may usefully respond to treatment with the following:**
A  metoclopramide
B  propranolol
C  phenytoin
D  carbamazetine
E  ergotamine

12.13 A **True**
B **True** more common than lipohypertrophy. Occurs to a lesser degree when the newer purified insulins are used
C **False** these occur as part of the immune process considered responsible for the development of insulin-dependent diabetes (type 1)
D **True** Insulin-induced hypoglycaemia may cause a number of symptoms and signs of central nervous system dysfunction: headache, blurred vision, mental confusion, coma and seizures
E **True** Insulin promotes $K^+$ uptake into cells by stimulation of the $Na^+$, $K^+$-ATPase enzyme system

12.14 A **False** although transient changes in liver enzyme concentrations and liver function tests have been reported they are not considered to be of any great clinical significance
B **False** cimetidine has rarely been associated with hepatotoxicity
C **True** a toxic effect of methyldopa is hepatitis, which usually appears within the first two months of treatment. It is usually reversible, but may progress to hepatic cirrhosis
C **True** up to 12% of patients on isoniazid may have elevated liver enzymes. Hepatic damage leading to cirrhosis is rarer and appears to be more common in older patients
E **True** hepatoxicity with salicylates appears to be dose-dependent and not due to a hypersensitivity reaction

12.15 A **False**
B **False** propranolol and metoclopramide have no place in the treatment of trigeminal neuralgia
C **True** may be useful in some cases not responding to treatment with carbamazepine
D **True** preferred drug. If taken during the acute stages of trigeminal neuralgia, reduces the frequency and severity of attacks
E **False** useful in the treatment of acute attacks of migraine

**12.16    Drugs useful in the management of hyperlipidaemia include**
A    cholestyramine
B    L-thyroxine
C    nicotinic acid
D    bezafibrate
E    vitamin E

**12.17    Hydralazine**
A    has no significant effect on heart rate
B    is subject to extensive first-pass metabolism by the liver
C    is useful in the treatment of hypertensive emergencies
D    may cause depression
E    can cause fluid retention

**12.18    Dipyridamole**
A    acts by inhibiting phosphodiesterase
B    should not be given with warfarin
C    increases the bleeding time
D    is useful in the treatment of migraine
E    causes postural hypotension

12.16 A **True**    useful in lowering LDL-cholesterol in conditions such as familial hypercholestecolaemia
      B **False**   dextrothyroxine has lipid lowering properties (LDL), but is associated with an increase in the frequency of angina in patients with ischaemic heart disease and is no longer recommended
      C **True**    treatment with nicotinic acid is associated with an early fall in triglyceride levels (VLDL) and a later fall in LDL-cholesterol
      D **True**    is indicated for the treatment of the following classes of hyperlipidaemia (Fredrickson): type IIa, IIb, III, IV and V
      E **False**   at the present time no therapeutic value has been found in any condition for vitamin E when used in man

12.17 A **False**   a compensatory tachycardia occurs following vasodilatation due to direct relaxation of arteriolar vascular smooth muscle
      B **True**    the extent of this metabolism depends on the acetylator status of the patient. 'Fast' acetylators metabolise the drug more quickly and tend not to experience side-effects to the same degree as 'slow' acetylators
      C **True**    hydralazine should be given intravenously with caution in hypertensive emergencies to reduce blood pressure quickly and to avoid unwanted hypotension
      D **False**   anxiety and sleep disturbances have been associated with the use of hydralazine, but depression is not a feature of treatment with this drug
      E **True**    by increasing renal blood flow, the renin-angiotensin-aldosterone system is stimulated and causes fluid retention

12.18 A **True**    this causes an increase in the level of intracellular AMP
      B **False**   although there is little evidence for a role in the treatment of stroke, transient ischaemic attacks or postoperative deep vein thrombosis, dipyridamole may be of benefit in combination with warfarin in patients with prosthetic heart valves
      C **False**   however, in vitro effects on platelet function have been demonstrated
      D **False**
      E **False**   in normal doses, dipyridamole has only slight effects on systemic blood vessels. It has been shown to dilate coronary arteries, but this effect has not been shown to be of clinical importance

**12.19  Alcohol (ethyl alcohol)**
  A  suppresses rapid eye movement sleep (REM)
  B  causes an increase in the NAD/NADH ratio following
       metabolism
  C  increases the secretion of antidiuretic hormone (ADH)
  D  is useful in the treatment of methyl alcohol poisoning
  E  causes a flushing reaction in patients taking
       chlorpromazine

**12.20  In acute intermittent porphyria**
  A  morphine is contraindicated
  B  convulsions can be treated with barbiturates
  C  hypertension can be treated with propranolol
  D  the symptoms and signs may resemble lead poisoning
  E  desferrioxamine infusion may be useful in the treatment of
       the acute attack

12.19 A **True**

B **False**    alcohol is mainly metabolised by cytosolic alcohol dehydrogenase using NAD as a coenzyme. Therefore the ratio NAD/NADH falls

C **False**    alcohol acts on the supraoptic nucleus of the hypothalamus to inhibit ADH secretion. This accounts in part for the polyuria following alcohol ingestion

D **True**    administration of alcohol depresses the rate of metabolism of methylalcohol preventing accumulation of toxic metabolites

E **False**    an alcohol-relating flushing syndrome is seen with chlorpropamide, a sulphonylurea hypoglycaemic agent, not with chlorpromazine

12.20 A **False**    drugs which may provoke an acute attack include: barbiturates, oral contraceptives, anticonvulsants, alcohol, sulphrylureas and sulphonamides

B **False**    barbiturates may exacerbate the condition (see answer to part A)

C **True**

D **True**    a predominantly motor peripheral neuropathy as in lead poisoning may develop during an acute attack

E **False**    desferrioxamine may be of benefit in treating the excess hepatic iron deposition seen in porphyria cutanea tarda.

# Chapter 13

**13.1** In a patient with mania the following treatment would be useful
- A haloperidol
- B prochlorperazine
- C oral high-dose diazepam
- D lithium carbonate
- E amitriptyline hydrochloride

**13.2** Ocular drug toxicity may be seen in the following circumstances
- A trimethoprim treatment of urinary tract infection
- B ethambutol treatment of tuberculosis
- C chloroquine in rheumatoid arthritis
- D depot phenothiazine treatment of schizophrenia
- E amiodarone treatment of Wolff-Parkinson-White syndrome

**13.3** In a patient with multiple myeloma the following drugs would be a useful treatment
- A melphalan
- B mithramycin if hypercalcaemia occurred
- C high-dose oral prednisolone if the patient had hypercalcaemia
- D acyclovir
- E azathioprine

**13.4** Erythema nodosum may be associated with the following drugs
- A the combined oestrogen-progestagen contraceptive pill
- B sulphonamide drugs
- C depot phenothiazine drugs
- D chlorpropamide
- E thiazide diuretics

13.1  A  **True**    also droperidol, both are butyrophenones
      B  **False**   is a phenothiazine used mainly as an antiemetic
      C  **False**   benzodiazepines have no place in mania
      D  **True**    for severe manic-depressive psychosis it is a good
                     drug; electroconvulsive therapy may also be used
      E  **False**   tricyclics are only of use for depression

13.2  A  **False**
      B  **True**    patients must be followed by an opthalmologist
      C  **True**    again, an opthalmologist must see the patient
                     regularly
      D  **False**
      E  **True**    lens opacities may occur

13.3  A  **True**    a 'standard' drug used for many years
      B  **True**    care: this antibiotic is nephrotoxic
      C  **True**
      D  **False**   an antiviral drug. However, who knows, for it has
                     been reported to benefit idiopathic aplastic anaemia
      E  **False**   used only in 'autoimmune' disorders

13.4  A  **True**    also it can occur in pregnancy — due, presumably, to
                     the high oestrogen state?
      B  **True**
      C  **False**
      D  **False**
      E  **False**

**13.5    In the disease/condition stated, the following drugs may be used to relieve pruritis**

A    cholestyramine in primary biliary cirrhosis
B    terfenadine in allergic uticaria
C    alcohol in pruritis associated with Hodgkin's disease
D    oral aluminium hydroxide in chronic renal failure
E    griseofulvin in scabies

**13.6    Cardiac failure may be exacerbated or precipitated by the following drugs**

A    metoclopramide
B    propranolol
C    metformin
D    minoxidil
E    indomethacin

**13.7    A patient presents with oedema and frothy urine; there is proteinuria of <5 g per day, hypocholesterolaemia, low plasma protein concentrations and raised serum creatinine concentrations. The following statements are true**

A    the patient has the nephrotic syndrome
B    indomethacin may stop the proteinuria
C    high-dose prednisolone may be beneficial
D    this syndrome may be a side-effect of the phenoxymethyl penicillin which the patient was taking
E    the condition could have been produced if the patient was epileptic and taking long-term carbamazepine

**13.8    A patient with generalised anxiety neurosis presents to her general practitioner; the doctor would be correct in recommending the following treatment**

A    six months treatment with lorazepam
B    an initial two weeks course of diazepam
C    six weeks treatment with amitriptyline
D    a course of psychotherapy and behaviour therapy
E    treatment with oral phenelzine

**13.9    An increased dose of insulin may be needed in a previously stable diabetic if the patient**

A    is entering the third trimester of pregnancy
B    develops chronic renal failure
C    has a severe streptococcal throat infection
D    has the insulin form changed from beef to a porcine monocomponent-type insulin
E    if the patient has hypertension treated with captopril

13.5  A **True**    or in any cholestatic jaundice by binding bile salts in
                    the gut, preventing their reabsorption and
                    accumulation in skin
      B **True**    terfenadine is a new $H_1$-antihistamine, less sedating
                    than conventional $H_1$-histamine antagonists
      C **False**   pruritis occurs in Hodgkin's and alcohol causes
                    flushing in Hodgkin's but does not affect the pruritis
      D **True**    possibly by binding phosphate
      E **False**

13.5  A **False**
      B **True**    beta-blockade decreases cardiac output
      C **False**
      D **True**    by causing vasodilatation increased renin secretion
                    and thereby hyperaldosteronism (added to that of
                    any cardiac failure) and salt and water retention
      E **True**    causes salt and water retention possibly by inhibiting
                    synthesis of natriuretic prostaglandins (it does not
                    work via renin the secretion of which it inhibits)

13.7  A **True**    do not forget there are many types
      B **True**    unknown mechanism
      C **True**    in minimal change type of glomerulonephritis
                    causing the nephrotic syndrome
      D **False**
      E **False**   occurs with phenytoin (also troxidone which used to
                    be used for petit mal)

13.8  A **False**   this would be relatively long-term treatment with a
                    benzodiazepine and lorazepam has been one of the
                    most-incriminated benzodiazepines as a cause of
                    dependence and withdrawal phenomena
      B **True**    this short initial course of benzodiazepine has its
                    length approved by the august body of the CSM!
      C **False**   this is indicated in withdrawn depression; it could
                    make the patient's agitation worse
      D **True**
      E **False**   a monoamine oxidase inhibitor would not be used
                    here, though they can be used for severe phobic
                    anxiety

13.9  A **True**    there is usually an increase in insulin requirement.
                    Patients should be hospitalised for careful diabetic
                    control
      B **False**   insulin sensitivity is increased in chronic renal failure
      C **True**    all infections may precipitate diabetic precoma
      D **False**   a reduction in dose is likely to be needed, if in doubt
                    we would admit the patient for the changeover
      E **False**

**13.10   Trigeminal neuralgia may conventionally be treated with the following**
A   phenytoin
B   long-term oral opiate analgesics
C   carbamazepine
D   phenol injection of the Gasserian ganglion
E   oral pizotifen prophylaxis

**13.11   In Ménière's disease the following drugs may be useful**
A   oral frusemide
B   betahistine
C   thiazide diuretics
D   chlorpropamide
E   intramuscular streptomycin

**13.12   Hypokalaemia is a recognised complication of**
A   long-term spironolactone treatment
B   use of combination tablets of amiloride and a thiazide diuretic to treat hypertension
C   acetazolamide therapy for glaucoma
D   chronic large doses of purgatives
E   long-term cimetidine maintenance treatment

**13.13   In acute infections of the paranasal sinuses the following treatment is appropriate**
A   oral amoxycillin
B   oral tetracyclines such as doxycycline
C   intranasal sodium chromoglycate
D   nasal ephedrine drops
E   oral nalidixic acid

**13.14   A patient complains to you of a chronic stuffy nose, he is hypertensive and treated with methyldopa and prazosin. He recently had coryza 4 weeks ago and since then has been using 'otrivine' (xylometazoline, an alpha-adrenoceptor agonist) nasal spray. The following statements are true about his condition**
A   methyldopa could be a cause of the stuffy nose
B   prazosin could be a cause of the stuffy nose
C   if his blood pressure had recently increased, xylometazoline could have contributed to this
D   the otrivine nasal spray should be stopped
E   his antihypertensive treatment needs review

13.10 A **False**
      B **False**    though in the past the pain has been so terrible that
                     these have been resorted to
      C **True**     initial treatment of choice
      D **True**     but causes corneal anaesthesia and so risks damage
      E **False**    a 5-HT antagonist for migraine prophylaxis

13.11 A **False**
      B **True**
      C **True**     may act by altering otolymph secretion
      D **False**
      E **False**    streptomycin may cause cochlear and/or vestibular
                     nerve damage

13.12 A **False**    this aldosterone antagonist may cause
                     hyperkalaemia
      B **True**     amiloride retains potassium but thiazides cause a
                     loss and their hypokalaemic effect may be dominant:
                     monitor plasma potassium (hyperkalaemia, too, may
                     occur due to amiloride especially with a degree of
                     renal failure)
      C **False**    due to inhibition of distal renal tubule carbonic
                     anhydrase potassium-sodium-hydrogen ion
                     exchange, hyperkalaemic acidosis may occur
      D **True**     a myopathy may occur presumably due to potassium
                     loss and melanosis coli — black colonic pigmentation
                     — and a typical barium enema appearance
      E **False**

13.13 A **True**     penetrates well into purulent exudates
      B **True**     good penetration to infected sinuses
      C **False**    only used for allergic rhinitis
      D **True**     as a decongestant to help unblock the sinus ostia
                     which may be covered by swollen mucosa: do not
                     use for longer than 2–3 days because of risk of
                     'rhinitis medicamentosa'
      E **False**    water-soluble 'antiseptic' used only in urinary tract
                     infections

13.14 A **True**     well-known side-effect
      B **True**     Also well-known — common with alpha-blockade
      C **True**     large doses with absorption through the mucosa
                     could produce this effect
      D **True**     he may have boggy, hyperaemic nasal mucosa
                     following prolonged use of a nasal decongestant
      E **True**     this is a strange combination; it would seem to run a
                     high risk of postural hypotension, for instance (both
                     drugs cause this)

**13.15  In a pregnant woman the fetus may be adversely affected under the following circumstances**

A  occasional maternal injection of paracetamol for headache
B  treatment of maternal epilepsy with phenytoin
C  treatment of maternal deep vein thrombosis and pulmonary embolus by heparin
D  treatment of maternal urinary tract infection with amoxycillin
E  treatment of maternal vomiting with a phenothiazine antiemetic

**13.16  The following antibiotics are appropriate for immediate treatment of the infections or conditions stated.**

A  erythromycin in campylobacter gastroenteritis
B  phenoxymethylpenicillin for hospital-acquired *E. coli* urinary tract infection
C  intravenous vancomycin to cover hip-replacement
D  oral vancomycin in *Clostridium difficile* pseudomembranous colitis
E  intravenous ampicillin + an aminoglycoside to cover urethral surgery in a patient with a heart valve defect

**13.17  In a patient receiving warfarin therapy**

A  the warfarin is largely plasma protein bound
B  alopecia may result from the warfarin
C  warfarin increases the risk of cardiac arrhythmias
D  the dose of warfarin will need adjustment if he develops atrial fibrillation and is treated with digoxin
E  the dose of warfarin may need to be decreased if he is given amiodarone

**13.18  A 55-year-old woman who is a smoker is admitted to hospital with a bout of severe retrosternal chest pain**

A  if the cause is peptic stomach ulcer pain, the antiulcer effect of cimetidine will be antagonised by her smoking
B  if she has a myocardial infarction, subsequent treatment with propranolol will decrease the risk of a reinfarction
C  if she has a pulmonary embolus then intravenous heparin should be given
D  if she has acute cholecystitis, pain relief is best given by intravenous diamorphine
E  if she has a pneumothorax, then an underwater seal drain should be inserted immediately

13.15 A **False** occasional paracetamol seems safe
  B **True** cleft palate may occur but treatment must be continued because of the risks of fits otherwise; also epilepsy is associated with a small increased risk of fetal malformations independent of anticonvulsants
  C **False** some mothers are maintained on subcutaneous heparin throughout pregnancy (stopped 24 h before parturition)
  D **False** penicillins are wonderfully safe
  E **True** phenothiazines localize in the developing uveal tract and may cause blindness or visual field defects

13.16 A **True** campylobacter cause mainly abdominal pain and diarrhoea — often bloody
  B **False** unless a culture shows sensitivity, but a 'hospital organism?' is likely to be resistant
  C **False** intravenous vancomycin is toxic. Fucidic acid and clindamycin could be used
  D **True** the infection is localized to the gut wall and the oral vancomycin acts locally and is not absorbed
  E **True** genitourinary manipulation has a high incidence of bacteraemia and cover should be given when there is a predisposition to infective endocarditis

13.17 A **True** hence the risk of displacement of warfarin and increased anticoagulant effects by some drugs
  B **True** this is a possible side-effect of all anticoagulants including heparin
  C **False**
  D **False**
  E **True** amiodarone is highly protein-bound and may displace warfarin This was difficult but amiodarone is being used increasingly to treat paroxysmal supraventicular tachycardia, so you may meet it in practice

13.18 A **True** reasoning 'a priori' but has also been shown in a clinical trial
  B **True** shown also for timolol, metoprolol and alprenolol
  C **True** for its immediate anticoagulant and (little-known) antiplatelet effects
  D **False** opiates, especially heroin and morphine, cause spasm of smooth muscle and, therefore, of the sphincter of Oddi. Pethidine is usually used for biliary colic, but we cannot understand why because it too causes smooth muscle spasm whereas phenazocine does much less so
  E **False** she should first be evaluated for degree of dyspnoea and (via chest X-ray) size of pneumothorax and presence of mediastinal shift

**13.19**   A 60-year-old woman with non-insulin-dependent diabetes mellitus presents with malaise and palpitations. Her blood potassium is 6.0 mmol/l, creatinine clearance 26 ml/min and plasma glucose 25 mmol/l. She has hypertension and is taking a combined tablet of propranolol and spironolactone (spiroprop) and glibenclamide for the diabetes

    **A**   the spiroprop should be stopped

    **B**   a thiazide diuretic would have been appropriate treatment for her hypertension

    **C**   the propranolol may have worsened her diabetic control

    **D**   she may need insulin treatment

    **E**   an angiotensin converting enzyme inhibitor (captopril or enalapril) would be useful to treat her hypertension

**13.20**   The following are effects or side-effects of digoxin therapy

    **A**   hypokalaemia

    **B**   disturbed blood glucose control

    **C**   xanthopsia

    **D**   inverted correction mark" change ('cupping') of the e.c.g. ST-segment

    **E**   gynaecomastia

13.19 A **True**    beta-antagonists and spironolactone retain
potassium and she is hyperkalaemic — maybe the
palpitations are symptomatic of the hyperkalaemia

   B **False**   this would have worsened her diabetes

   C **True**    propranolol and other beta-antagonists do this as
well as masking and blocking compensatory
mechanisms for hypoglycaemia

   D **True**    her diabetes is poorly controlled but her propranolol
should first be stopped and compliance with diet and
glibenclamide checked before insulin is given;
combination of glibenclamide with metformin should
probably be tried before resorting to insulin

   E **False**   these cause potassium retention

13.20 A **False**

   B **False**

   C **True**    seeing yellow or green-yellow colours

   D **True**    usually taken as a sign of 'digoxin-effect' when seen
in leads with a dominant R wave, but if present
throughout all e.c.g. leads may be a sign of early
digoxin toxicity

   E **True**

# Chapter 14

**14.1** It is important to monitor the responses of the following drugs as indicated in each case below

A heparin by prothrombin time
B warfarin by whole blood clotting time
C lithium carbonate by plasma drug concentration
D theophylline in children by salivary drug concentration
E nifedipine by plasma drug concentration

**14.2** A 75-year-old woman presents with an offensive vaginal discharge and vulval irritation. A diagnosis of atrophic vaginitis is made. Drugs of use in her management would be

A a single intramuscular high dose of a depot penicillin
B vaginal clotrimazole pessaries and clotrimazole vulval cream
C the oral contraceptive pill
D topical vulval oestrogen cream
E oral preparation of equine-conjugated oestrogens

**14.3** In systemic lupus erythematosis (SLE)

A the patient may respond to high-dose prednisolone
B a combination of mustine, vincristine, prednisolone and procarbazine would be useful
C use of azathioprine would enable a smaller dose of prednisolone to be used
D hyperbaric oxygen therapy may be helpful
E penicillamine may stop disease progression

**14.4** In a patient with scabies, correct treatment would be

A topical antihistamine ointment to decrease pruritis
B oral terfenadine to decrease pruritis
C twice daily topical gamma-benzene hexachloride
D topical Whitfield's ointment to the lesions
E twice daily topical application of DDT

14.1  A **False**  heparin is an antithrombin and so invalidates prothrombin time, therefore use whole blood clotting times

B **False**  warfarin, of course, is monitored by prothrombin time

C **True**  though here you are guarding against a toxic response rather than guaging a therapeutic response

D **True**  salivary concentration is roughly equivalent to free (i.e. non-plasma protein-bound) theophylline concentration

E **False**

14.2  A **False**  this is used for gonorrhoea; most unlikely here

B **True**

C **False**  thromboembolic and fluid retention risks

D **False**

E **True**  less risk of thromboembolic phenomena than synthetic oestrogens

14.3  A **True**  initial treatment of choice but tail off rapidly to as small a maintenance dose as possible

B **False**  this is used for Hodgkin's disease

C **True**

D **False**  not used. Hyperbaric oxygen has been largely discredited for multiple sclerosis treatment recently

E **False**  it may modify rheumatoid progression, but does not affect SLE

14.4  A **False**  topical antihistamines are little used now because they may sensitise the skin and produce allergic eruptions

B **True**  a new less-sedating histamine $H_1$-antagonist

C **True**  the drug known as 'gammexane' or 'quellada'

D **False**  only used for ringworm and pityriasis

E **False**  toxic

**14.5**  **The following features would be attributed to propranolol in a non-insulin-dependent diabetic patient who is taking the drug for hypertension:**
   A   prolongation of the cephalin-kaolin (partial thromboplastin) time
   B   breathlessness on exercise
   C   severe nightmares
   D   muscle pain
   E   increased glycosylated haemoglobin concentration

**14.6**  **Interferon**
   A   is produced naturally in certain virus-infected cells
   B   may be used for treatment of hairy-cell leukaemia
   C   can be given orally for prophylaxis of coryza
   D   may cause an influenza-like syndrome as a side-effect (fever, chills, headache, malaise, myalgia)
   E   may cause bone marrow suppression

**14.7**  **You are asked what you would recommend for the treatment of a young schizophrenic. The following drugs would be likely to be of use in ameliorating the schizophreniform symptoms**
   A   phenelzine
   B   flupenthixol
   C   long-term dexamethasone
   D   regular intramuscular fluphenazine undecanoate
   E   droperidol

**14.8**  **Acyclovir**
   A   is a natural product of human cells which have been infected with certain viruses
   B   can be given topically to decrease the intensity of herpes labialis
   C   can be given intravenously to prevent dissemination of varicella-zoster virus in immunodeficient patients
   D   when given intravenously, decreases the pain and increases rate of healing of varicella-zoster lesions
   E   is effective in decreasing the duration of symptoms of the common cold

14.5   A  **False**
       B  **True**     due to decreased cardiac output, cardiac failure could
                       occur
       C  **True**     propranolol crosses the blood-brain barrier — lipid
                       soluble beta-blockers seem to cause bad dreams
       D  **True**     usually only on high doses
       E  **True**     beta-antagonists impair glucose control in type II
                       diabetics possibly by preventing insulin secretion
                       (partially beta-receptor-mediated)

14.6   A  **True**     there are many types of interferon. Interferon as a
                       'drug' is made from human leucocyte cultured cell
                       lines or by recombinant nucleic acid techniques in
                       bacteria
       B  **True**     the only indication for which interferon has a product
                       license in Britain
       C  **False**    is protein therefore destroyed by gut secretions
       D  **True**
       E  **True**     blood count must be monitored, can also cause
                       abnormal liver function tests

14.7   A  **False**   this is a monoamine oxidase inhibitor for depression
       B  **True**     a thioxanthene with properties like the
                       phenothiazines
       C  **False**
       D  **True**     A depot phenothiazine
       E  **False**    this is one of the butyrophenones which are used for
                       mania

14.8   A  **False**   do not confuse with interferons
       B  **True**
       C  **True**
       D  **True**
       E  **False**

**14.9**  A patient aged 59 took diazepam for 5 years, but a psychiatrist tells the general practitioner to stop the diazepam since the patient is depressed but not anxious. The general practitioner stops the diazepam immediately and the patient is given amitriptyline. Two days later the patient has anxiety, myoclonic jerks, paraesthesiae, tachycardia, a feeling of walking on cottonwool and his blood pressure is 140/90 sitting and 80/40 on standing

   A   the general practitioner should not have stopped the diazepam suddenly

   B   the postural hypotension resulted from stopping the diazepam

   C   amitriptyline could have been a factor in causing the postural hypotension

   D   the amitriptyline unmasks the patient's anxiety

   E   intravenous phenytoin is indicated in this patient

**14.10**  The following points are true with regard to intravenous infusions

   A   the site of a long-term infusion should be changed regularly to prevent thrombophlebitis

   B   particulate matter in the infusion may be excluded by using a filter in the infusion line

   C   use of glass ampoules for infusion additives may result in the intravenous injection of glass particles

   D   most long-term infusions should be given in dextrose, in preference to saline, because there is less risk of thrombophlebitis with dextrose than saline

   E   insulin infusions into an intravenous line via a filter may not deliver the whole dose of the insulin added to the infusate

**14.11**  In a patient who is otherwise well but complains of insomnia

   A   increase in alcohol intake may cure the problem

   B   a milk and cereal drink, e.g. Horlicks, at bedtime improved sleep

   C   oral chlorpromazine would be an appropriate hypnotic

   D   occasional temazepam at night can be permitted for treatment of insomnia

   E   prolonged use of a benzodiazepine hypnotic may result in rebound insomnia when the drug is stopped

14.9  A **True**      the patient has benzodiazepine withdrawal
                    phenomenon, all the described symptoms are
                    common in this; fits and opistothonus may occur
      B **False**
      C **True**     a well-known side-effect of amitriptyline
      D **False**
      E **False**    the patient has myoclonus, not full blown epilepsy; a
                    benzodiazepine, clonazepam (cf. *CLONus*) is often
                    used for myoclonus

14.10 A **True**      probably at least every 24–48 hours
      B **True**      modern methods of manufacture have lessened the
                    degree of particulate contamination but it still occurs
      C **True**      fragments may be aspirated into the syringe used for
                    drawing up the drug (read for yourself in *British
                    Medical Journal* 1985, 291: 1390)
      D **False**     dextrose (glucose) given intravenously has a
                    tendency to cause thrombophlebitis
      E **True**      insulin adsorbs onto filters; another drug which
                    commonly does so is vincristine sulphate

14.11 A **False**     alcohol intake should be limited (inital stimulant
                    effect, increased urinary frequency)
      B **True**      proven by science! (See *Sleep* 1980, 3: 47)
      C **False**     this phenothiazine would not be appropriate in an
                    otherwise well patient
      D **True**      regular use should be discouraged because of
                    tolerance then rebound after drug withdrawal;
                    however, banning use of benzodiazepine hypnotics
                    would seem inhumane
      E **True**      possibly also associated with deep REM sleep and
                    dreaming

**14.12    In establishing an intravenous cannula for intravenous infusion of drugs**

A    a small intradermal injection of lignocaine locally may decrease the pain of cannula insertion

B    if the first attempt fails and the needle is partially withdrawn through the cannula, the needle must not be reinserted for another attempt at venepuncture

C    a tourniquet should not be used because it increases the chance of extravasation of blood if venepuncture fails

D    use of the filter in the line may decrease risk of subsequent thrombophlebitis

E    after cannula insertion the arm must, in every case, be immobilised in splint to prevent disconnection of the cannula

**14.13    A patient is hypertensive but is well-controlled on propranolol. He complains of dyspepsia and is given oral magnesium hydroxide. A week later his doctor found that the patient's blood pressure had increased. Therefore**

A    magnesium hydroxide is likely to have a direct vasoconstrictor effect and elevates blood pressure

B    the patient may have diarrhoea subsequent to taking magnesium hydroxide

C    the prescription of magnesium hydroxide may have caused the increase in blood pressure

D    if the dyspepsia persists, enteric-coated aspirin would be an appropriate analgesic to relieve the dyspeptic pain

E    if the dyspepsia persists then cimetidine would be useful in relieving the pain

**14.14    5-hydroxytryptamine antagonists are useful in the following situations**

A    ketanserin to prevent flushing in the carcinoid syndrome

B    methysergide to treat retroperitoneal fibrosis

C    ketanserin to treat essential hypertension

D    ketanserin for treatment of migraine

E    methysergide for petit mal epilepsy

**14.15    The following can be direct effects of alcohol (ethanol)**

A    an increased mean corpuscular volume

B    facial flushing in a patient who is taking metronidazole

C    acute tubular necrosis in a patient taking a tetracycline drug

D    alopecia

E    cerebral atrophy

14.12 A **Don't** a double-blind clinical trial has not been done but the
      **know** clinical impression is that lignocaine works in this
             respect
      B **True** reinsertion might fragment the cannula tip with entry
             of particles into the circulation
      C **False** a tourniquet is useful or a sphygmomanometer (cuff
             inflated but below diastolic pressure) in difficult cases
      D **True** since a filter excludes particles which seem to
             increase risk of thrombophlebitis
      E **False** securing the cannula and a tap to the skin with
             simple adhesive is usually all that is needed

14.13 A **False** one cannot conclude this from the observation made
      B **True** cf. aluminium hydroxide which constipates
      C **True** antacids may decrease absorption of propranolol and
             a number of other drugs, including iron, and if the
             antacid contains calcium, tetracyclines
      D **False** non-steroidal anti-inflammatory drugs would be
             contraindicated in case a peptic ulcer is the cause of
             the dyspepsia
      E **True** histamine $H_2$-antagonists are good for relieving
             dyspepsia, but a diagnosis of the cause *must* be
             made

14.14 A **True** due to 5HT-2 receptor antagonism
      B **False** retroperitoneal fibrosis is a serious side-effect of
             methysergide used for prophylaxis of migraine
      C **True** a recently revealed use of the drug
      D **True**
      E **False**

14.15 A **True** presumably a combination of direct marrow toxicity
             and decreased folate intake in the usually poor diets
             of heavy drinkers
      B **True** so-called 'antabuse effect'
      C **False**
      D **False**
      E **True** a common finding in heavy drinkers. Alcohol may
             cause many central nervous system syndromes —
             look them up some time!

**14.16** A hospitalised 72-year-old woman complains of polyuria; she has occasional dizziness when she walks in the ward and she has been treated for cardiac failure with bumetanide

A   a blood glucose estimation would be of value in managing this patient
B   the dose of bumetanide should be reviewed
C   she may be hyperkalaemic due to the bumetanide
D   if culture of the patient's urine shows a growth of *E. coli* then this is likely to be sensitive to phenoxymethyl penicillin
E   the patient's lying and standing blood pressure should be measured

**14.17** A 56-year-old non-insulin-dependent diabetic taking glibenclamide has essential hypertension. The following may be true in management of his conditions

A   the initial treatment of choice for his hypertension would be a thiazide diuretic
B   atenolol would be contraindicated
C   spironolactone might exacerbate his diabetes
D   a calcium antagonist such as verapamil or nifedipine would not worsen his diabetes
E   it would be important to measure his renal function

**14.18** An 80-year-old patient who has had cardiac failure and hypertension treated with moduretic (combination of hydrochlorthiazide and amiloride) presents with slight confusion and upper motor neurone signs in the legs; his plasma sodium is 121 mmol/litre. The following are true of this patient's condition

A   the neurological signs in the legs and confusion could be due to hyponatraemia
B   the low plasma sodium may have been caused by the moduretic
C   his plasma potassium needs checking
D   the moduretic should be stopped and his cardiac status reviewed
E   he is likely to be more sensitive to hydrochlorthiazide or amiloride than a patient aged 40 years

14.16 A **True**    the lady may have diabetes mellitus (idiopathic or
bumetanide-induced)
  B **True**    she may need a smaller dose or none at all and
bumetanide may be causing postural hypotension or
dizziness due to a cardiac arrhythmia resulting from
hypokalaemia
  C **False**    but she may well be hypokalaemic
  D **False**    it would be likely to be resistant since it probably will
be hospital-acquired; her urine should be cultured,
for infection may cause polyuria
  E **True**    she may have exercise postural hypotension as the
cause of her dizziness

14.17 A **False**    thiazide diuretics impair glucose tolerance
  B **False**    beta-antagonists have the theoretical risk of masking
hypoglycaemic symptoms and impairing glucose
mobilisation from the river (a $beta_2$- adrenergic
response). In practice, many diabetics have been
treated without problems with a beta-antagonist
  C **False**    this is one of the indications for using spironolactone
to treat hypertension (but watch hyperkalaemia
especially in renal failure)
  D **True**    these are useful drugs for treating hypertension in
diabetcis
  E **True**    because both diabetes and hypertension could cause
renal damage, which would increase risk of drug
side-effects such as prolonged hypoglycaemia from
glibenclamide, or, if atenolol was used (B above),
might impair its excretion so causing excessive
bradycardia (atenolol has a long action and
undergoes mainly renal excretion)

14.18 A **True**    the plasma sodium is very dangerously low and
could cause confusion, but other causes must also be
investigated
  B **True**    hyponatraemia has been well-documented with
combinations of a thiazide and distal tubular diuretic
in elderly patients; if you prescribe these
combinations you must monitor patients' electrolytes
  C **True**    hyperkalaemia (due to the amiloride) and
hypokalemia (due to the thiazide) have been
described with combinations of thiazides and
potassium-sparing diuretics
  D **True**    when in doubt, stop the drug!
  E **True**    a fact well-known to geriatricians but not so well by
other physicians

**14.19** An 82-year-old man is given imipramine for incontinence and is also taking 'madopar' (combination of L-dopa + dopa-decarboxylase inhibitor) for parkinsonism. He has attacks of dizziness on standing up from his chair and says his vision is too blurred to read his paper. The following are true

A   he may have postural hypotension due to imipramine
B   he may have postural hypotension due to the madopar
C   the use of L-dopa alone without a decarboxylase inhibitor would be safer for this patient
D   stopping the imipramine may cure his blurred vision
E   imipramine increases the risk of tardive dyskinesia due to the madopar

**14.20** In a patient with diabetes mellitus, it is true that

A   strict control of blood glucose correlates with decreased incidence of complications
B   human insulin is superior to monocomponent porcine insulin for treatment of diabetes
C   treatment with an aldose reductase inhibitor may decrease the risk of some diabetic complications
D   treatment of atrial fibrillation with digoxin may destabilise the control of the diabetes
E   treatment of cardiac failure with bumetamide may aggravate the diabetes

14.19 A **True**   imipramine has been used as an experimental model
                   for postural hypotension — always suspect it
      B **True**   postural hypotension is well-documented for L-*dopa*
      C **False**  there is no evidence for this and the reverse should
                   be true for the decarboxylase inhibitor decreases
                   peripheral metabolism of L-dopa to dopamine and
                   so decreases the risk of cardiac arrhythmias
      D **True**   blurred vision may be due to the postural
                   hypotension but, if persistent, is more likely to be
                   due to the anticholinergic ciliary body paralysis
                   caused by imipramine; patients may become tolerant
                   to this
      E **False**  to our knowledge!

14.20 A **True**
      B **False**  there is no evidence for superiority of human over
                   monocomponent insulin, even though the
                   manufacturers would wish it so
      C **True**   you are up to date if you got this one! Aldose
                   reductase, by converting glucose to the sugar alcohol
                   galactitol, may be involved in genesis of diabetic
                   microangiopathy
      D **False**
      E **True**   bumetanide, a loop diuretic, may exacerbate diabetes
                   mellitus

# Chapter 15

**15.1** **The following drugs should be used with caution in the clinical situations described**

    **A** tetracyclines in chronic renal failure
    **B** nitrofurantoin in G6PD deficiency
    **C** gentamicin in myasthenia gravis
    **D** metronidazole in ulcerative colitis
    **E** amoxycillin in pulmonary embolism

**15.2** **Are the following statments true or false**

    **A** bicarbonate does not enhance the excretion of amphetamine
    **B** fatty food reduces the absorption of griseofulvin
    **C** probenecid slows the excretion of indomethacin
    **D** the absorption of amoxycillin is considerably greater than that of amipicillin
    **E** flucloxacillin is a more potent antistaphylococcal penicillin than cloxacillin

**15.3** **If the effects on blood pressure of drug A are compared with drug B in a clinical trial and there is a significant difference at the 5% level**

    **A** there is a 5% chance that these drugs really do have a different effect on blood pressure
    **B** the power of the study is such that there is a 95% chance of detecting a difference if one exists
    **C** this result could have occurred by chance with a probability of 1 in 20
    **D** a type II error could not account for this finding
    **E** this suggests that the more efficacious drug would be of use clinically

15.1   A **True**   when renal function is impaired tetracyclines may
                      cause renal toxicity
       B **True**   along with many other drugs, may cause haemolysis
       C **True**   applies to the other aminoglycosides too
       D **False**  may be given safely when the differential diagnosis
                      includes pseudomembranous colitis
       E **False**  no increase in toxicity or loss of efficacy

15.2   A **True**   renal amphetamine excretion is enhanced when the
                      urine pH is acid
       B **False**  fatty food increases its absorption
       C **True**   together with several other drugs, e.g. penicillin and
                      acyclovir
       D **True**   serum concentrations after amoxycillin approach
                      twice those after ampicillin
       E **False**  absorption of flucloxacillin is more extensive, but
                      potency is similar

15.3   A **False**  there is a 95% chance that there is a real difference
       B **False**  no information about the power of the study was
                      given
       C **True**   conversely, there is a 95% chance this result did not
                      occur by chance
       D **True**   a type II error occurs when a no difference result
                      occurs when a difference exists and a type I error
                      occurs when a significant difference occurs by
                      chance
       E **False**  a statistical difference does not imply a biologically
                      significant difference

**15.4    In a clinical trial**

A    double blind means that investigator and subject should not be allowed to see the treatment

B    a crossover study means that all subjects should receive all treatments

C    a parallel group study means that subjects should receive each treatment at the same time as other subjects

D    a Latin square design means that subjects receive each treatment in every combination of orders

E    a controlled study means that subjects all receive placebo as well as another treatment

**15.5    When analysing the results of a clinical trial**

A    a paired t test will give an idea of the correlation between two variables

B    an analysis of variance can be used to identify the effect of treatment on peak expiratory flow rates in a study population

C    where a population characteristic is not distributed normally (such as blood pressure) a non-parametric statistical test must be used to test an hypothesis relating to the effect of treatment on that characteristic

D    when the mean, median and mode coincide, the distribution of a variable is normal

E    a chi square test could be used to identify a preponderance of fetal malformations in a drug-treated group of pregnant women compared with a control group

**15.6    The following foodstuffs should be prohibited to patients taking monoamine oxidase inhibitors:**

A    peanut butter

B    Marmite

C    cheese

D    chicken liver

E    yoghurt

**15.7    Lead poisoning may cause**

A    normochromic normocytic anaemia

B    basophilic stippling of red cells

C    wrist and foot drop

D    elevated delta amino laevulinic acid (DALA) hydratase in urine

E    abdominal pain

15.4   A **False**   the treatments should appear the same
       B **True**
       C **False**   each group receives the same treatment as others within the group but different from subjects in other groups
       D **False**   each treatment is given an equal number of times but not all possible orders of treatments are represented. A balanced Latin square design implies all treatment orders are represented equally
       E **False**   the control treatment is not necessarily placebo but may be an active drug

15.5   A **False**   the test identifies differences in means whereas correlation analysis identifies the relationship between two variables
       B **True**    particularly useful when more than two treatments have been given
       C **False**   if the distribution can be normalised, e.g. by a logarithmic transformation, a parametric analysis can be used
       D **True**
       E **True**    suitable for testing frequency differences between nominal groups

15.6   A **False**
       B **True**    the main danger is tyramine, an indirectly acting sympathomimetic normally metabolised by monoamine oxidase
       C **True**
       D **True**
       E **False**

15.7   A **True**    due to erythroid hypoplasia
       B **True**    due to deposits of lead within the red cells
       C **True**    other motor nerves less susceptible and sensory nerves not affected
       D **False**   this enzyme is sensitive to lead and its activity in blood is markedly reduced. This increases DALA in the urine
       E **True**    abdominal X-rays may also show opacities in the bowel

**15.8    Self poisoning with drugs**
- A    is more common in men than women
- B    constitutes at least 25% of emergency medical admissions to hospital under the age of 30 years
- C    is more likely to be a manifestation of psychiatric illness in older patients than younger patients
- D    frequently involves the ingestion of more than one drug
- E    is only rarely associated with the consumption of alcohol

**15.9    Gynaecomastia may result from treatment with the following drugs**
- A    phenothiazines
- B    methyldopa
- C    barbiturates
- D    digoxin
- E    prednisolone

**15.10    The following drugs or classes of drugs cause vasodilatation**
- A    slow calcium channel blockers
- B    methyldopa
- C    angiotensin converting enzyme inhibitors
- D    alpha$_1$ blockers
- E    non-selective beta blockers

**15.11    In a patient unconscious from self poisoning**
- A    small pupils suggest benzodiazepines as the cause
- B    pupil size is often helpful in suggesting barbiturate intoxication
- C    supportive management rather than the use of antidotes is the most important determinant of a successful outcome
- D    seizures caused by tricyclic antidepressants may respond to intravenous physostigmine
- E    a blood alcohol level is often helpful

15.8   A  **False**
       B  **True**
       C  **True**     because of this difference in aetiological factors,
                       older patients frequently have a genuine desire to kill
                       themselves rather than merely to seek attention
       D  **True**
       E  **False**    common association, presumably a reflection of the
                       widespread use of alcohol as well as the notion that
                       the effects will be additive

15.9   A  **True**     effect on hypothalamus producing
                       hyperprolactinaemia
       B  **True**     also hyperprolactinaemic effect
       C  **False**
       D  **True**     oestrogen-like effect
       E  **False**    no sex steroid activity

15.10  A  **True**     otherwise known as calcium channel blockers, these
                       agents have a variety of actions including relaxation
                       of vascular smooth muscle
       B  **False**    methyldopa, like clonidine, acts centrally to reduce
                       sympathetic outflow via central alpha agonism
       C  **True**     these agents, among other actions, reduce circulating
                       angiotensin II concentrations, thus withdrawing a
                       powerful vasoconstrictor
       D  **True**     peripheral alpha$_1$ blockers, e.g. prazosin and
                       indoramine, produce vasodilatation
       E  **False**    beta$_2$ *agonists* are vasodilators

15.11  A  **False**    benzodiazepines rarely cause unconsciousness and
                       in any event do not affect pupil size
       B  **False**    barbiturates, although an important cause of
                       unconsciousness, have a variable effect on pupil size
       C  **True**     most deaths relate to the complications of
                       unconsciousness rather than the specific toxic effects
                       of drugs
       D  **True**     however, this measure should be reserved for
                       serious complications because of the risk of
                       cholinergic overstimulation
       E  **True**     unconsciousness in a patient smelling of alcohol with
                       only a moderate blood alcohol concentration must be
                       due to some other cause

**15.12  Dosage reduction is necessary when prescribing the following drugs for the elderly**
- A  thiazide diuretics
- B  loop diuretics
- C  digoxin
- D  gentamicin
- E  atenolol

**15.13  The following drugs may cause bone marrow depression**
- A  gold salts
- B  radioactive iodine
- C  intravenous contrast media
- D  thiouracil
- E  chloramphenicol

**15.14  The following drugs are aldehyde dehydrogenase inhibitors**
- A  metronidazole
- B  sulphonylureas
- C  disulfiram
- D  paraaminosalicylic acid
- E  theophylline

**15.15   The following drugs may cause peripheral neuropathy**
- A  ethambutol
- B  nitrofurantoin
- C  insulin
- D  isoniazid
- E  prednisolone

**15.16  The following drugs may cause hyperuricaemia**
- A  thiazide diuretics
- B  alcohol
- C  pyrazinamide
- D  enalapril
- E  sulphinpyrazone

**15.17  The following drugs may cause hepatic toxicity**
- A  halothane
- B  pyrazinamide
- C  phenothiazines
- D  methotrexate
- E  ethambutol

15.12 A **False**
    B **True**     symptoms of postural hypotension are the main danger
    C **True**     hence the value of the 0.0625 mg tablets
    D **True**     like digoxin, gentamicin is renally excreted and physiological reduction of glomerular filtration occurs with advancing years
    E **False**

15.13 A **True**     hence the value of monitoring platelet counts
    B **False**
    C **False**
    D **True**     carbimazole is less toxic
    E **True**     worldwide, the most common cause of drug-induced aplastic anaemia

15.14 A **True**     hence the need for abstention from alcohol during treatment
    B **True**     probably less potent inhibitor than metronidazole
    C **True**     this activity is the desired effect of the drug
    D **False**
    E **False**

15.15 A **False**     at the high doses originally used in the treatment of TB, optic neuritis was a complication of therapy with this drug
    B **True**     fortunately a rare complication
    C **False**
    D **True**     seen only in slow acetylators and can be prevented by coadministration of pyridoxine
    E **False**     may, however, cause a myopathy

15.16 A **True**     all diuretics have this effect
    B **True**     elevated serum uric acid concentrations are common among chronic alcohol abusers
    C **True**     this drug is becoming more widespread in the treatment of TB. Its hyperuricaemic effect is due to its main metabolite pyrazinoic acid
    D **False**
    E **False**     this drug is uricosuric

15.17 A **True**     hepatic necrosis is a very rare complication usually after repeated administration
    B **True**     due to hepatitis
    C **True**     due to cholestasis. This reaction is idiosyncratic, not dose related
    D **True**     due to hepatic fibrosis
    E **False**

**15.18　In treating patients with hypertension the following may produce unacceptable hypotension**

A　captopril given to a patient on a diuretic
B　the first dose of prazosin
C　sublingual nifedipine
D　intravenous diazoxide
E　sodium nitroprusside

**15.19　Diarrhoea may be associated with the following drugs**

A　verapamil
B　magnesium trisilicate
C　aluminium hydroxide
D　ampicillin
E　codeine

**15.20　Amenorrhoea may be caused by the use of**

A　tricyclic antidepressants
B　combined oral contraceptives
C　beta blockers
D　H$_2$ blockers
E　phenothiazines

15.18 A **True**   diuretics should ideally be stopped before starting an
                   angiotensin converting enzyme inhibitor
    B **True**   the first dose should be taken after retiring to bed
    C **True**   the absolute fall in blood pressure after this drug is
                   related to the height of the starting pressure
    D **True**   the old regimen of 300 mg given by rapid i.v.
                   injection is dangerous and should no longer be used.
                   If oral therapy with other drugs cannot be used,
                   repeated miniboluses of 50 mg appear safe
    E **True**   must be given by i.v. infusion with very careful
                   continuous blood pressure monitoring

15.19 A **False**   causes constipation
    B **True**   magnesium-containing antacids may all cause
                   diarrhoea
    C **False**   aluminium and calcium-containing antacids may
                   cause constipation
    D **True**   all broad-spectrum antibiotics may do this
    E **False**   all the opiate derivatives tend to cause constipation

15.20 A **True**   due to hyperprolactinaemia
    B **True**   only if taken continuously
    C **False**
    D **False**
    E **True**   due to hyperprolactinaemia

# Chapter 16

**16.1** **The following drugs cross the placenta and may be hazardous to the fetus**

    **A** warfarin
    **B** radioiodine
    **C** thiouracil
    **D** propranolol
    **E** heparin

**16.2** **The following antibiotics act by interfering with bacterial protein synthesis**

    **A** phenoxymethylpenicillin
    **B** erythromycin
    **C** cotrimoxazole
    **D** nystatin
    **E** griseofulvin

**16.3** **The following antibiotics are bacteriostatic**

    **A** Penicillins
    **B** erythromycin
    **C** cotrimoxazole
    **D** isoniazid
    **E** chloramphenicol

**16.4** **The following drugs are indicated in acute severe asthma**

    **A** sodium cromoglycate
    **B** atropine
    **C** adrenaline
    **D** antibiotics
    **E** mucolytics

**16.5** **The following drugs undergo significant presystemic metabolism after oral administration**

    **A** theophylline
    **B** glyceryl trinitrate
    **C** hydralazine
    **D** labetalol
    **E** nadolol

16.1  A **True**  in the first trimester warfarin may be teratogenic. At delivery warfarin may cause dangerous uterine bleeding
    B **True**  administration of both drugs is also incompatible with
    C **True**  breast feeding
    D **False**  Beta-blockers are safe in pregnancy
    E **False**  Heparin does not cross the placenta

16.2  A **False**  act on the cell wall
    B **True**
    C **False**  both sulphonamides and trimethoprim are folate antagonists
    D **False**  acts on the cell membrane
    E **False**  interfere with nucleic acid metabolism

16.3  A **False**
    B **True**
    C **False**  sulphonamides alone, however, are bacteriostatic
    D **False**
    E **True**

16.4  A **False**  only indicated for prophylaxis of attacks
    B **False**  the value of the inhaled ipratropium bromide (also an antimuscarinic agent) is, however, controversial
    C **False**  selective beta$_2$ agonists should now be used
    D **False**  antibiotics should be reserved for bacterial infections which may coexist in a minority of cases
    E **False**  these agents have never been shown to be beneficial

16.5  A **False**  low hepatic extraction ratio. Bioavailability virtually 100%
    B **True**  hence it is given sublingually or transdermally
    C **True**  as a result the bioavailability may be as low as 8% in some fast acetylators
    D **True**  as with other drugs, there is marked intersubject variability in the extent of presystemic metabolism
    E **False**  cleared by the kidneys

**16.6    In a patient with a creatinine clearance of 25 ml/min**

    **A**   the normal dose of cimetidine should be reduced
    **B**   propranolol should be avoided altogether
    **C**   the dose of amoxycillin should be reduced
    **D**   isoniazid at normal dosage is safe
    **E**   dextropropoxyphene may produce c.n.s. toxicity

**16.7    In a patient with moderately impaired liver function (e.g. due to cirrhosis)**

    **A**   atenolol would be entirely safe
    **B**   dosage reduction of verapamil would be wise
    **C**   the risk of lactic acidosis due to metformin therapy is increased
    **D**   idiosyncratic hepatic reactions to drugs would be more common
    **E**   theophylline containing preparations should be prescribed at normal dosage

**16.8    Antacids may reduce the extent of absorption of**

    **A**   isoniazid
    **B**   theophylline
    **C**   pivampicillin
    **D**   tetracyclines
    **E**   cimetidine

**16.9    The following drugs may impair driving performance**

    **A**   caffeine
    **B**   methyldopa
    **C**   amphetamine-like drugs
    **D**   amitriptyline
    **E**   beta-agonists

**16.10  Monoamine oxidase inhibitors**

    **A**   may have a beneficial effect in Parkinson's disease
    **B**   should not be prescribed for a patient who cannot abstain from alcohol
    **C**   can safely be prescribed without a special diet in patients taking hypotensive medication
    **D**   may be selective with sparing of monoamine oxidase in the gut
    **E**   may be useful in treating neuroses

**16.11  Pyridostigmine**

    **A**   crosses the blood-brain barrier
    **B**   is indicated in the prophylaxis of malaria
    **C**   may increase salivary volume
    **D**   when given i.v. forms the basis of a test for myasthenia gravis
    **E**   interacts with theophylline

16.6  A **True**    to avoid confusional state and deterioration in renal function
      B **False**   almost all of the metabolic products of propranolol are inactive and their accumulation will not produce clinical effects
      C **False**   only necessary in severe renal failure (creatinine clearance < 10 ml/min)
      D **True**    dosage reduction necessary only in severe renal failure
      E **True**    due to accumulation of metabolites

16.7  A **True**    renally excreted
      B **True**    higher blood concentrations result from dosing by any route
      C **True**    this was particularly important with phenformin before it was taken off the market
      D **False**   only dose-related hepatic reactions are more common in patients with hepatic impairment
      E **False**   dosage reduction is necessary

16.8  A **True**
      B **False**
      C **True**
      D **True**    due to chelation
      E **True**    dosing of the antacid and cimetidine should be separated by an hour to avoid this interaction

16.9  A **False**   indeed, it produces central nervous stimulation which may increase alertness
      B **True**    sedative effect in many patients
      C **True**    increased risk-taking behaviour
      D **True**    particularly early on in treatment
      E **False**

16.10 A **False**   increasing local dopamine concentrations
      B **True**    many alcoholic drinks also contain tyramine
      C **False**   the cheese reaction remains dangerous
      D **True**    selegiline is a type B MAOI which is safe without a diet
      E **False**   should be reserved for patients with psychotic depression

16.11 A **False**   physostigmine is the only anticholinesterase drug that crosses the blood–brain barrier
      B **False**
      C **True**    cholinergic effect
      D **False**   this is the 'Tensilon' or edrophonium test
      E **False**

**16.12    The following drugs dilate the pupil**
    **A**  phenylephrine
    **B**  topical beta blockers (e.g. timolol)
    **C**  tropicamide
    **D**  pilocarpine
    **E**  dexamethasone

**16.13    The following drugs can lower intraocular pressure**
    **A**  cyclopentolate
    **B**  atropine
    **C**  propranolol
    **D**  acetazolamide
    **E**  chloramphenicol

**16.14    The following drugs can be detected in breast milk in significant amounts after maternal administration**
    **A**  rifampicin
    **B**  theophylline
    **C**  isoniazid
    **D**  atenolol
    **E**  nadolol

**16.15    The efficacy of the following drugs is reduced in renal failure**
    **A**  hypotensive drugs
    **B**  probenecid
    **C**  nitrofurantoin
    **D**  cotrimoxazole
    **E**  cimetidine

**16.16    The following drugs can be used to lower serum cholesterol without long-term risks**
    **A**  nicotinic acid
    **B**  clofibrate
    **C**  cholestyramine
    **D**  propranolol
    **E**  colestipol

**16.17    Chenodeoxycholic acid**
    **A**  will bind bile acids in the gut
    **B**  frequently causes diarrhoea
    **C**  is useful in dissolving gall stones as long as they contain some cholesterol
    **D**  is metabolised to ursodeoxycholic acid
    **E**  may take many months to dissolve gall stones

16.12 A **True**    alpha₁ agonist
      B **False**
      C **True**    anticholinergic
      D **False**   constricts pupil due to cholinomimetic effect
      E **False**

16.13 A **False**   may increase intraocular pressure due to
                    anticholinergic effect
      B **False**   long-acting anticholinergic effect
      C **True**    all beta-blockers will do this. Due to reduced aqueous
                    production
      D **True**    due to carbonic anhydrase inhibition reducing
                    aqueous production
      E **False**

16.14 A **True**    probably does the baby no harm, however
      B **True**    rarely has effects on the baby
      C **True**    hence the baby should be given pyridoxine to
                    prevent the development of peripheral neuropathy
      D **False**
      E **True**    hence atenolol is preferred

16.15 A **True**    due to salt and water retention
      B **True**    allopurinol, however, remains effective but dosage
                    reduction is necessary to avoid toxicity
      C **True**    poor urine penetration
      D **False**   however, trimethoprim alone in reduced dosage
                    should be used to avoid toxicity
      E **False**   again dosage reduction is needed to avoid toxicity

16.16 A **True**    facial flushing after dosing is a problem. Also
                    biochemical adverse effects
      B **False**   effective agent but associated with an excess of large
                    bowel malignancies
      C **True**    many patients find it unpleasant to take
      D **False**   beta-blockers have no beneficial effect on cholesterol
                    or lipids and may have a deleterious effect
      E **True**    like cholestyramine, acts by binding bile acids. The
                    long-term effects are not yet known but to date
                    appears safe

16.17 A **False**
      B **True**    this makes ursodeoxycholic acid a better alternative
      C **False**   stones must be well visualised on cholecystography
                    and contain no calcium
      D **True**    this agent seems equally effective
      E **True**    hence this therapy is not suitable for patients with
                    frequent or severe complications of gall stones

**16.18  In ulcerative colitis**

  A   steroids are useful in prophylaxis of acute episodes
  B   sulphasalazine is useful in prophylaxis of acute episodes
  C   sulphasalazine may be substituted by 5-amino salicyclic acid
  D   arthritis and chronic active hepatitis are indications for steroid therapy
  E   bulk laxatives may be needed to control constipation

**16.19  When prescribing a tricyclic antidepressant**

  A   imipramine would be a good choice in a patient in whom sedation would be undesirable
  B   amitriptyline has little sedative action
  C   all agents have some anticholinergic action
  D   coexistent epilepsy is not a contraindication
  E   postural hypotension may result

**16.20  When the following pairs of drugs are precribed together a pharmacodynamic drug interaction would be expected**

  A   beta-agonists and methyl xanthines
  B   oestrogen and warfarin
  C   cimetidine and propranolol
  D   isoniazid and phenytoin
  E   prazosin and verapamil

16.18 A **False**  helpful only in the treatment of relapses
      B **True**   also of help in mild attacks when an increased dose
                   may be helpful
      C **True**   this is the most active component and is useful in
                   patients unable to tolerate sulphasalazine.
                   Sulphasalazine toxicity is more common in slow
                   acetylators as the sulphapyridine component is
                   metabolised by acetylation
      D **True**   as are many other systemic manifestations
      E **True**   particularly during the early phase of remission when
                   diseased segments may not allow faeces to pass
                   through

16.19 A **True**   may sometimes have a c.n.s. stimulating effect
      B **False**  marked sedation
      C **True**   a non-tricyclic such as mianserin would be more
                   appropriate
      D **False**  may often lower epileptic threshold
      E **True**   due to weak alpha$_1$-blocking activity

16.20 A **True**   producing increased bronchodilatation
      B **True**   oestrogens reduce the anticoagulant effect of
                   warfarin without affecting the prothrombin time
      C **False**  pharmacokinetic interaction — cimetidine increases
                   the bioavailability of propranolol
      D **False**  pharmacokinetic interaction — isoniazid inhibits the
                   metabolism of phenytoin
      E **True**   both are antihypertensives but, in addition, oral
                   verapamil will increase the AUC of oral prazosin,
                   hence there is also a pharmacokinetic interaction

# Chapter 17

**17.1** A patient was found to have a low level of serum thyroxine and thyroid stimulating hormone, serum tri-iodothyronine was also low. The following are true with regard to this patient

A the patient has primary hypothyroidism
B treatment should be started with L-thyroxine
C treatment should eventually be started with prednisolone, fludrocortisone and L-thyroxine
D treatment should be started with D-thyroxine
E blood should be taken for a repeat determination of thyroid function tests

**17.2** Genetically-engineered human insulin

A should be stored frozen at −70° Celsius
B carries a small but finite risk of transmitting the human immunodeficiency virus, the cause of AIDS
C may cause tingling in the hands, feet or tongue, together with sweating and dizziness if given in overdose
D is likely to be less antigenic than beef pancreas-derived insulin
E if stored in a refrigerator in the longer acting forms, may be cloudy in appearance but still active.

**17.3** A patient aged 20 years with cystic fibrosis has a cough with green sputum; *Pseudomonas* species are isolated from the sputum, but you are awaiting results of sensitivity tests. The following are true of this patient's management

A chest physiotherapy is contraindicated in this patient in case of causing rib fractures
B cefotaxime should be given in high doses by mouth
C intravenous erythromycin is an appropriate antibiotic
D oral ciprofloxacin may be of benefit
E intravenous carbenicillin could cure the chest infection

17.1  A  **False**  it is likely to be secondary hypothyroidism because serum TSH is low, reflecting possible pituitary or even hypothalmic malfunction

B  **False**  if pituitary of hypothalmic disease is present, then treatment of hypothyroidism without steroid cover could precipitate an Addisonian crisis

C  **True**  if diagnosis of secondary or tertiary hypothyroidism is made

D  **False**  D-isomers of amino acids and their derivatives are active only in bacteria and plants, not in animals

E  **True**  the diagnosis is so important that one needs to exclude any chance of laboratory measurement error before further tests are done to confirm disturbance of the hypothalamico-pituitary-thyroid or adrenal axis

17.2  A  **False**  freezing denatures insulin, it should be stored at +4°C in a refrigerator

B  **False**  human insulin is produced by bacterial action and then purified; there is no risk of AIDS' but patients may want to be assured of this, so you need to know the answer!

C  **True**  these are all symptoms of hypoglycaemia

D  **True**  beef insulin has many impurities present genetically-engineered insulin is identical to insulin made in the body; the preparative chromatographic techniques purify out all significant traces of bacterial protein (down to about 4 parts per million)

E  **True**  the cloudiness is due to binding of insulin to other substances in the mixture; only soluble insulin is clear

17.3  A  **False**  rubbish, chest physiotherapy with postural drainage of secretions is of vital importance in the management of these people who are now living much longer than in the past

B  **False**  cefotaxime does work against *Pseudomonas* but is not active by mouth

C  **False**  not active against *Pseudomonas*.

D  **True**  the first orally-active antipseudomonal antibiotic

E  **True**  one of the first antipseudomonal penicillins, Ticarcillin with or without clavulanic acid and aztreonam are also active parenterally against *Pseudomonas*

**17.4    The following drugs can be used to treat infections with the anaerobic organism *Bacteroides***

A    trimethoprim
B    metronidazole
C    amoxycillin and Clavulanic Acid (augmentin)
D    gentamicin
E    phenoxymethylpenicillin

**17.5    Immunoglobulins may be used in treatment of disease as follows**

A    as prophylaxis against hepatitis A (infectious hepatitis)
B    to treat digoxin toxicity
C    to treat paracetamol toxicity
D    to treat paraquat poisoning
E    to decrease incidence of side-effects from certain cytotoxic drugs

**17.6    The following drugs may be useful in the treatment of urgency incontinence**

A    diclofenac
B    terodiline
C    dicyclomine
D    imipramine
E    baclofen

**17.7    In a patient with bronchial asthma**

A    salbutamol should be inhaled regularly, four times a day, to prevent attacks occurring
B    inhaled budesonide decreased the number of acute attacks
C    inhaled beclomethasone decreases the number of acute attacks
D    inhaled terbutaline may relieve the bronchospasm of an acute attack
E    an oral theophylline preparation must always form an integral part of maintenance treatment

17.4   A  **False**
      B  **True**    best known drug for this
      C  **True**    not so well-known, but the combination is as
                   effective as metronidazole
      D  **False**
      E  **False**

17.5   A  **True**
      B  **True**
      C  **False**   methionine or cysteamine are used
      D  **False**   dialysis may be used in addition to supportive
                   measures
      E  **True**    using monoclonal antibodies to neoplasms, drugs
                   conjugated to these (an example is etoposide) may
                   be targeted at the neoplasms, so decreasing
                   exposure of the normal organs to the drugs

17.6   A  **False**   diclofenac is a non-steroidal anti-inflammatory drug
      B  **True**    this is a new anticholinergic and calcium antagonist
                   drug which acts by both these mechanisms to damp
                   down bladder muscle contractions in urgency
                   incontinence
      C  **True**    due to its anticholinergic effect
      D  **True**    due to its anticholinergic effect
      E  **False**   this is a gamma-aminobutyric acid agonist which
                   decreases spasticity.

17.7   A  **False**   beta-agonists are used only to relieve bronchospasm,
                   not for prophylaxis (this is often not known and it is
                   fortunate and interesting that asthmatics do not
                   seem to become tolerant to inhaled salbutamol or
                   terbutaline)
      B  **True**
      C  **True**
      D  **True**
      E  **False**   they should only be used as a last resort, their use
                   routinely makes it difficult to use intravenous
                   theophylline in a severe attack not relieved
                   sufficiently by nebulized bronchodilators. In truth,
                   this area is controversial: some physicians dislike i.v.
                   theophylline because of its central effects and prefer
                   i.v. beta-agonists. A bad question, but at least you
                   know both sides of the story?

**17.8**    You see a 68-year-old woman in the outpatient clinic; she has three ischaemic toes in each foot. The femoral, popliteal and foot pulses are palpable. The following points are true of this patient

A   the sustained release propranolol she is taking should be stopped immediately in the clinic

B   the dose of dipyridamole she is taking should be increased to increase blood flow into her feet

C   she should be put on conventional formulation propranolol and then she should be gradually weaned off this drug

D   her urine should be tested for glucose

E   she should be asked if her fingers turn cold and white when exposed to cold weather

**17.9**    The following are true of a patient in severe congestive heart failure due to ischaemic heart disease

A   oxygen therapy is contraindicated because it may cause depression of respiration

B   addition of an angiotension-converting enzyme inhibitor to the treatment may be beneficial

C   frusemide should be given at night so that diuresis may be maximal when the patient is lying in bed, so increasing renal blood flow

D   addition of a thiazide may be beneficial, even when the patient is taking a high dose of frusemide

E   isosorbide dinitrate or mononitrate may be of further benefit in a patient already receiving frusemide and captopril

**17.10**   A patient of 60 years of age has a left-sided hemiparesis due to a right-sided cerebrovascular accident, you presume. The patient has a blood pressure of 180/105 when seen first on the ward. The following are true of this patient's management

A   Glycerol may be beneficial treatment

B   The hypertension should be treated immediately

C   If the patient is on warfarin, a computerised tomographic scan should be arranged as soon as possible

D   If the patient is on warfarin, simultaneous treatment of a chest infection with erythromycin may have been responsible for the cerebrovascular accident

E   Oral drugs should be immediately replaced by parenteral preparations

17.8  A **False**  she could get a beta-blocker withdrawal syndrome with tachycardia, palpitations, angina and even myocardial infarction

B **False**  there is no evidence that dipyridamole helps peripheral vascular disease

C **True**  see answers to A above; conventional propranolol allows smaller decreasing doses to be given before stopping the drug

D **True**  her large blood vessels are clinically unaffected so she could have diabetic microangiopathy

E **True**  she might have Raynaud's phenomenon secondary to the propranolol, or to some other cause

17.9  A **False**  do not confuse with cor pulmonale

B **True**  there are studies showing that this decreased mortality rates

C **False**  renal blood flow is greater when people lie flat but frusemide given at night will not permit them to spend a long time lying flat without rising to respond to the diuresis!

D **True**

E **True**  higher doses of nitrates will decrease afterload so decreasing the need for cardiac work; the pro-drug dinitrate, or its active mononitrate metabolite, may be used

17.10 A **True**  has been shown repeatedly in clinical trials to be of benefit on a population basis, presumably by decreasing cerebral oedema around the injured areas

B **False**  we do not have enough information about strokes in general to know what to do about hypertension of this degree (it is different for malignant hypertension, in any case the blood pressure may decrease over the subsequent 24 hours

C **True**  in case of a subdural haematoma

D **True**  erythromycin potentiates the action of warfarin, an effect seen too often by one of the authors — look up interactions when prescribing for a patient on warfarin or phenindione

E **False**  the patient may be able to swallow well, but the gag reflex must always be checked in case of a bulbar component to the CVA (most often it is not checked it seems to one of the authors!)

**17.11** **Tricyclic antidepressants are known to possess the following pharmacological properties**

A   block neuronal uptake of 5-hydroxytryptamine (5-HT)
B   decrease rapid-eye-movement (REM) sleep
C   stimulate muscarinic cholinergic receptors
D   cause postural hypotension
E   shorten intracardiac impulse conduction

**17.12** **Phase IV (postmarketing surveillance) studies are designed to provide the following**

A   approval by the appropriate governing body to market the drug
B   new indications for prescribing a particular drug
C   pharmacokinetic data in healthy volunteers
D   drug efficacy in long-term use
E   idiosyncratic reactions to the drug (if any)

**17.13** **The following drugs were withdrawn from routine use in the United Kingdom because of the toxicity stated**

A   phenformin — lactic alkalosis
B   thalidomide — agranulocytosis
C   practolol — pleural fibrosis
D   benoxaprofen — fatal liver damage
E   phenylbutazone — digital gangrene

**17.14** **Diltiazem**

A   is a new angiotensin-converting enzyme (ACE) inhibitor
B   has a negative inotropic effect
C   is effective in relieving angina
D   should be given in reduced doses in the elderly
E   because of its long half-life must be given once daily

17.11  A  **True**
      B  **True**
      C  **False**    antagonism occurs, causing anticholinergic side
                      effects such as a dry mouth, blurred vision,
                      constipation, urinary retention, etc.
      D  **True**
      E  **False**    prolongs conduction time. Treatment with tricyclic
                      antidepressants may be associated with ventricular
                      arrhythmias, especially in patients who have pre-
                      existing heart disease

17.12  A  **False**    approval has already been given
      B  **True**
      C  **False**    this data is obtained from healthy volunteers during
                      phase 1 studies
      D  **True**
      E  **True**    unfortunately, a particular idiosyncratic reaction or
                      serious side-effect may only manifest itself after
                      thousands of patients have been treated with the
                      drug

17.13  A  **False**    phenformin was withdrawn from the United
                      Kingdom market because of its association with lactic
                      acidosis (not alkalosis). Metformin, the only
                      biguanide in common use, is said to be 15–50 times
                      less likely to cause lactic acidosis
      B  **False**    thalidomide was given to pregnant mothers for use
                      as a hypnotic, but was shown to cause major fetal
                      limb abnormalities (phocomelia)
      C  **True**    practolol was also shown to cause fibrosis of the eye,
                      pericardium, retroperitoneal tissues and skin
                      (oculomuco-cutaneous syndrome)
      D  **True**    other side effects reported included gastrointestinal
                      haemorrhage, thrombocytopenia, renal damage,
                      photosensitivity and eye toxicity
      E  **False**    aplastic anaemia and agranulocytosis complicate
                      treatment with phenylbutazone. Other serious side
                      effects, such as peptic ulcer, hepatitis, nephritis, etc.,
                      can occur in up to 10% of cases

17.14  A  **False**    diltiazem is a calcium-channel antagonist
      B  **True**    although this effect is less than for verapamil
      C  **True**    by virtue of its vasodilating effects on the coronary
                      and peripheral circulation and by reducing the heart
                      rate
      D  **True**
      E  **False**    diltiazem has a half-life of 3–4 h, which is prolonged
                      in elderly patients and after repeated administration

**17.15** **The following combinations of drugs have the potential to interact adversely**

  A  levodopa and reserpine
  B  cholestyramine and nicotinic acid
  C  carbamazepine and indomethacin
  D  amphetamine and ascorbic acid
  E  insulin and chlorpropamide

**17.16** **Isoprenaline**

  A  is a pure alpha-receptor agonist
  B  causes bronchodilatation
  C  produces a rise in mean blood pressure when given as an intravenous infusion
  D  has a metabolic fate similar to adrenaline
  E  should not be given in pregnancy

**17.17** **The following drugs may undergo abnormal metabolism in some patients due to genetic variation**

  A  metformin
  B  primaquine
  C  isoniazid
  D  penicillin
  E  suxamethonium

17.15 A **True**  reserpine can cause a Parkinsonian-like syndrome and would counteract the therapeutic benefit of levodopa

B **False**  these drugs act in synergism to reduce low-density lipoprotein (LDL) levels, which are, for example, raised in patients with familial hypercholesterolaemia

C **True**  both drugs may cause fluid retention (exact mechanism in either case unknown) and could potentially precipitate heart failure in patients with ventricular dysfunction

D **False**  interestingly, however, ascorbic acid can be used (as can ammonium chloride) to acidify the urine in patients with amphetamine poisoning, to facilitate renal excretion of this basic drug

E **True**  both drugs may predispose the patient to unwanted hypoglycaemia. However, trials are currently in progress in this country and in the United States to assess the usefulness (if any) of combining insulin with a sulphonylurea in patients with diabetes mellitus

17.16 A **False**  its actions are predominantly stimulatory on all beta-receptors, with only weak actions at alpha receptors

B **True**  by stimulation of beta-2 receptors

C **False**  although the cardiac output may rise and lead to an increase in systolic blood pressure, lowering of peripheral vascular resistance occurs and leads to a fall in mean blood pressure

D **True**

E **False**  the drug has been given in pregnancy. Data from animal studies has not shown any evidence of teratogenesis

17.17 A **False**  metformin does not undergo any appreciable metabolism

B **True**  in patients with glucose-6-phosphate dehydrogenase deficiency (a sex-linked recessive disorder), primaquine causes red blood cells to lyse (haemolysis)

C **True**  isoniazid is metabolised by acetylation. Slow acetylators are homozygous for a recessive gene, which puts them at a higher risk of developing peripheral neuropathy, which is a well-recognised side-effect of isoniazid therapy

D **False**

E **True**  about 1 in 3000 patients given suxamethonium become apnoeic. This is due to an abnormal variant of plasma cholinesterase which fails to hydrolyse acetylcholine, resulting in continued depolarisation at the muscle motor end plate

**17.18  The following statements referring to aluminium and its compounds are true**

A   aluminium chloride has mild antiseptic properties
B   aluminium hydroxide causes diarrhoea
C   chronic ingestion of aluminium-containing compounds may lead to osteomalacia
D   blood tetracycline levels are higher in patients receiving aluminium compounds
E   aluminium may cause meningitis

**17.19  Recognised side-effects of treament with minoxidil are**

A   alopecia
B   fluid retention
C   bradycardia
D   Steven-Johnson syndrome
E   hypertension

**17.20  Etidronate disodium (a diphosphonate)**

A   activates bone resorption
B   causes hypercalcaemia
C   is used to relieve pain in Paget's disease of bone
D   is not effective orally
E   may cause loss of taste

17.18 A **True**    aluminium is a constituent of some deodorant and
                    antiperspirant aerosols
      B **False**   causes constipation
      C **True**    in patients with normal renal function, aluminium-
                    induced phosphate-binding in the gastrointestinal
                    tract leads to bone-resorption and a negative calcium
                    balance. In patients with chronic renal failure, an
                    additional effect on bone mineralisation may occur
      D **False**   tetracyclines are chelated by aluminium compounds
                    and consequently are poorly absorbed from the
                    gastrointestinal tract
      E **False**   some cases of encephalopathy were seen in patients
                    with chronic renal failure and were found to be due
                    to aluminium, which was present as a contaminant in
                    the dialysis fluid

17.19 A **False**   Minoxidil has actually been employed to treat certain
                    cases of alopecia by virtue of its ability to cause
                    hypertrichosis
      B **True**    probably by increasing proximal tubule reuptake of
                    filtered sodium
      C **False**   causes a reflex tachycardia due to its vasodilating
                    action
      D **True**    this is a rare complication of treatment with this drug
      E **False**   blood pressure has a tendency to fall with minoxidil
                    because of its vasodilating action

17.20 A **False**   inhibition of bone resorption occurs. This process
                    may be related to inhibition of hydroxyapatite crystal
                    dissolution and/or a direct effect on the activity of
                    osteoclasts
      B **False**   etidronate has been used to treat hypercalcaemia
                    associated with malignancy
      C **True**    double-blind studies have shown diphosphonates to
                    be superior to placebo in relieving pain due to
                    Paget's disease of bone
      D **False**   however, absorption from the gastrointestinal tract is
                    poor with a bioavailability of only about 5%
      E **True**    transient changes in taste sensation have been
                    reported following use of the intravenous
                    preparation

# Chapter 18

**18.1 Sulphasalazine**
A is a useful treatment for rheumatoid arthritis
B is contraindicated in patients with inflammatory bowel disease
C may be replaced by mesalazine for the treatment of ulcerative colitis
D may cause systemic lupus erythematosus as a side-effect
E can cause a macrocytic anaemia

**18.2 The following drugs may be of use in the treatment of hypertrophic obstructive cardiomyopathy**
A digoxin
B amiodarone
C frusemide
D verapamil
E propranolol

**18.3 The following may be used to treat constipation in the elderly**
A rectal loperamide
B oral golytely
C sulphasalazine
D phosphate enemas
E oral sodium picosulphate plus magnesium citrate (picolax)

**18.4 In a patient presenting with a ventricular tachycardia, appropriate treatment may include**
A atropine intravenously
B oxygen
C intravenous lignocaine
D alternating current cardioversion
E insertion of an emergency temporary cardiac pacemaker

18.1   A **True**    increasingly recognised over the past 10 years
       B **False**   used to treat ulcerative colitis
       C **True**    mesalazine is a new alternative for patients who
                     cannot tolerate sulphasalazine
       D **False**
       E **True**    sulphasalazine may impair folate absorption and
                     hence cause a macrocytic anaemia

18.2   A **False**   might worsen the condition by increasing force of
                     contraction and hence increasing ventricular outflow
                     tract obstruction
       B **False**
       C **True**    if cardiac failure occurs, frusemide would be useful
       D **True**    Verapamil has been shown to decrease afterload and
                     decrease ventricular force of contraction
       E **True**    the decrease in force of contraction reduces the
                     outflow tract obstruction

18.3   A **False**   Loperamide is an antidiarrhoeal
       B **True**    this is a mixture of electrolytes which, when taken in
                     large volumes (beware of cardiac failure), may be
                     useful in resistant constipation and faecal impaction
       C **False**
       D **True**    any enema is likely to clear the rectum
       E **True**    picolax is a powerful cathartic and is much used in
                     bowel-preparation for radiological/endoscopic
                     studies; powerful cathartics may be dangerous in
                     faecal impaction where there is a risk of bowel
                     perforation

18.4   A **False**   atropine speeds the heart by its anticholinergic
                     activity
       B **True**
       C **True**
       D **False**   synchronised direct current cardioversion
       E **False**   overdrive pacing would not be performed at
                     presentation unless other measures had failed

**18.5**    **An elderly diabetic man has abnormal liver function tests, raised serum urea and creatinine, a deep penetrating ulcer over one heel and is on glibenclamide 10 mg daily. The following statements are true**

A    stopping glibenclamide may result in the liver function tests returning to normal
B    a change of treatment to insulin may increase the chance of the foot ulcer healing
C    glibenclamide is a likely cause of renal failure
D    an X-ray of the foot may lead to prescription of flucloxacillin and fusidic acid
E    there is minimal risk of hypoglycaemia from the glibenclamide

**18.6**    **A 75-year-old man has prostatic carcinoma with bony secondaries; he could be given, appropriately, the following treatments**

A    testicular gamma radiation
B    oestradiol plus a progestagen orally
C    goserelin by subcutaneous depot injection
D    oral stilboestrol
E    oral bromocriptine

**18.7**    **An outpatient is on a diabetic diet and has lost weight. He was diagnosed diabetic 2 years previously, with a fasting glucose of 4 mmol/l and values at 30, 60, 90 and 120 minutes of 8.4, 10.4, 7 and 5 mmol/l respectively; at the time of diagnosis he was taking methyldopa and prednisolone, currently he takes only methyldopa. The following statements about this patient are correct**

A    he should be given insulin
B    he should be prescribed a sulphonylurea
C    the glucose tolerance test should be repeated
D    his glycosylated haemoglobin should be measured, then the diabetic diet stopped and the glycosylated haemoglobin repeated after 3 months
E    prednisolone may have caused the abnormal glucose tolerance test

**18.8**    **The following statements about pharmacokinetics are true**

A    the half-life of penicillin is about 20 minutes
B    indomethacin and ibuprofen both have long half-lives and can be given twice daily
C    frusemide is predominantly excreted via the kidneys
D    the dose of gentamicin, rather than the dose interval, should be reduced in renal failure
E    aspirin shows non-linear pharmacokinetics

18.5   A **True**   sulphonylureas may cause hepatotoxicity
     B **True**   his diabetes may be better controlled on insulin
     C **False**
     D **True**   he may have osteomyelitis, for which these antibiotics would be appropriate; fusidic acid gives good penetration to bone and both have antistaphyloccal activity
     E **False**   there is an appreciable risk. For this reason the short-acting tolbutamide would have been a preferable agent

18.6   A **False**   he could have a surgical orchidectomy
     B **False**
     C **True**   this is a new LHRH analogue given subcutaneously every month it produces a 'medical orchidectomy'
     D **True**   it has oestrogenic side-effects including deep venous thrombosis. Cyproterone acetate (an antiandrogen, but not an oestrogen) is an effective alternative
     E **False**

18.7   A **False**
     B **False**
     C **True**   the original mildly diabetic glucose tolerance test with normal (below 5) fasting glucose concentration may have been due to the effect of prednisolone
     D **True**   glycosylated haemoglobin will give an idea of long-term blood glucose control. The repeat after stopping the diet should be at 3 months to allow 'wash out' of haemoglobin in red cells circulating at the time he was on his diabetic diet (red cell life 120 days)
     E **True**   a dose-related phenomenon

18.8   A **True**   hence the need for 2–4 hourly i.v. injections of penicillin in life-threatening infections such as meningitis
     B **False**   both need to be given three times daily
     C **True**   it only exerts its effects from within the renal tubules
     D **False**   the dose is determined by the volume of distribution whereas the dosing interval is determined by clearance which is reduced in renal failure
     E **True**   the rapid metabolism of aspirin to salicylate and the subsequent metabolism of salicylate are both saturable

18.9    A 20-year-old female presents with fever, sore throat, palpable
        cervical lymph nodes and splenomegaly; you are worried that
        the sore throat is due to a bacterial infection but feel that she
        may have infectious mononucleosis. Your management of this
        patient may correctly include

        A    prescription of amoxycillin in case the sore throat is caused
             by bacterial infection
        B    paracetamol for the fever
        C    erythromycin to cover any bacterial cause of the sore
             throat
        D    a monospot test
        E    serological tests for syphilis

18.10   A patient with secondary carcinomatous bony deposits in the
        spine complains of severe back pain. The pain could be
        relieved by

        A    combination of a non-steroidal anti-inflammatory drug and
             paracetamol
        B    calcitonin
        C    regular twice daily doses of sustained-release morphine
             sulphate
        D    oral etidronate
        E    an intramuscular depot phenothiazine

18.11   An acute pancreatitis may occur due to the following
        conditions

        A    treatment with enteric-coated prednisolone
        B    treatment with intramuscular chlorpromazine
        C    in a patient taking oral bendrofluazide (a thiazide diuretic)
        D    in a patient with hypothermia
        E    during treament with methyldopa

18.12   The following therapies may sometimes be effective in
        relieving the pain of postherpetic neuralgia

        A    carbamazepine
        B    chlorpromazine
        C    trigeminal nerve block
        D    transcutaneous nerve stimulation
        E    intravenous acyclovir

18.9  A **False**  if she has glandular fever then she has a very high chance of having a rash with amoxycillin or ampicillin

B **True**

C **True**  erythromycin provides similar antibacterial cover to penicillins (but is also effective against *Legionella*, *Chlamydia* and certain other pathogens) and is not associated with a rash in glandular fever patients. The need for an antibiotic should be carefully considered

D **True**  to obtain a rapid diagnosis of glandular fever

E **False**  false positive serology may result during glandular fever

18.10  A **True**  a commonly used and useful combination

B **False**  only of use for pain in Paget's disease of bone

C **True**  a very useful formulation of morphine once the pain has been controlled and the necessary dosage defined with conventional morphine

D **False**  useful only for pain in Paget's disease of bone

E **False**  depot preparations are only used in patients with psychoses for long-term management. I.m. preparations are to be avoided in patients with terminal illnesses in view of their unpleasant nature. Phenothiazines by other routes may be useful adjuncts in such patients

18.11  A **True**  steroids have been associated with pancreatitis

B **False**

C **True**  All thiazides have this very rare risk

D **True**  Recognised complication

E **False**  Other drugs capable of causing pancreatitis are alcohol and azathioprine

18.12  A **True**

B **False**

C **True**

D **True**  also true of stimulation of the affected spinal segment with a vibrator

E **False**  oral or intravenous acyclovir ameliorates the attack but seems to have no effect on the incidence or the pain of postherpetic neuralgia

**18.13   The following drugs may prevent the thrombotic complications of atherosclerosis**

   A   dihomo-gammalinolenic acid
   B   nifedipine
   C   enalapril
   D   eicosapentaenoic acid
   E   low-dose aspirin

**18.14   The following items were included in a single prescription by a doctor: sulphasalazine 500 mg t.d.s. for 365 days and colifoam (foam containing hydrocortisone acetate 10%) b.d. for 365 days The pharmacist would be correct in the following**

   A   he should dispense the drugs as written
   B   he suggests that the duration of treatment is too long
   C   he thinks that the patient is likely to have ulcerative colitis
   D   he is correct in asking the doctor to write 'three times' and 'twice', 'daily' instead of respectively 'tds' and 'bd'
   E   he asks for the doses of the drugs used and the amount prescribed to be written in words as well as figures

**18.15   A patient with Parkinson's disease takes carbidopa plus L-dopa at 06.00, 1400, 1800 hours, but experiences marked rigidity and hypokinesia after each dose. Manoeuvres which may help the patient include**

   A   adding neostigmine to the treatment
   B   giving extra doses between the four stated times
   C   adding phenelzine to the treatment
   D   adding selegiline to the treatment
   E   trying a low-protein diet

18.13 A **True**
     B **False**
     C **False**
     D **True**
     E **True**

     *Note.* Aspirin in low doses prevents platelet aggregation by inhibiting platelet thromboxane synthetase but not prostacyclin synthetase, so that platelet aggregation caused by thromboxanes can be prevented while the antiplatelet aggregation effects of vessel wall prostacyclin are not prevented (high-dose aspirin inhibits vessel wall prostacyclin synthetase too). Dihomogammalinolenic acid and eicosapentaenoic acid divert prostaglandin synthesis to anti-thrombotic derivatives, they are found in oil of evening primrose and oily fish respectively. Eicosapentaenoic acid made from fish oils has been marketed. The fish are probably tastier!

18.14 A **False**
     B **True**    this encourages the patient not to be assessed by his doctors and is unsafe. Colifoam contains a large amount of topical steroid and should not be prescribed continually for 1 year without supervison
     C **True**
     D **True**    as recommended in the British National Formulary
     E **False**   words as well as figures and the exact number of tablets/volumes to be prescribed is necessary only for controlled drugs

18.15 A **False**   neostigmine is an anticholinesterase and hence could have the opposite effect to that required
     B **True**    a recognised method of combating L-dopa tolerance and the on-off phenomenon
     C **False**   this is dangerous because it can cause severe hypertension
     D **True**    selegiline is a selective monoamine oxidase type B inhibitor (unlike phenelzine) and dose not cause hypertension when combined with L-dopa preparations
     E **True**    certain amino acids interfere with L-dopa L-(dihydroxyphenyl alanine) absorption and reducing the competitive effects of these amino acids in foods may increase response to L-dopa

**18.16**   A patient with chronic obstructive airways disease is admitted with an infective exacerbation, he has been taking salbutamol and ipratropium inhalers and had been started on prednisolone and erthyromycin four days previously by his general practitioner. The patient was also taking warfarin following a femoral embolectomy 2 years previously. His international normalised Prothrombin ratio (INR) was 7.0 on admission. Correct management of this patient would include

    A   prescription of nebulised salbutamol and ipratropium
    B   vitamin K together with prednisolone
    C   increase in dose of erythromycin
    D   blood taken for grouping and saving of serum for transfusion if needed
    E   treatment with intravenous protamine sulphate

**18.17**   In the Stevens-Johnson syndrome with erythema multiforme

    A   treatment with a sulphonamide may have been the cause
    B   intravenous acyclovir is indicated
    C   topical corticosteoid ointment is needed
    D   corticosteroid should be given systemically
    E   treatment of a streptococcal sore throat with penicillin may have caused the syndrome

**18.18**   A hospital patient is treated for cardiac failure and diabetes mellitus with bendrofluazide and tolbutamide; her blood uric acid is raised but she has no joint pains. Prophylactic indomethacin is started. The following are true of this patient

    A   the indomethacin should be stopped
    B   tolbutamide may have contributed to the hyperuricaemia
    C   stopping the bendrofluazide may decrease the level of hyperuricaemia
    D   she should be given potassium supplements or a potassium-retaining diuretic
    E   her urea and electrolytes and body weight should be monitored

**18.19**   In the treatment of the irritable bowel syndrome

    A   sulphasalazine is useful maintainance treatment
    B   mebeverine may relieve the abdominal pain
    C   rectal steroid enemas are a recognised treatment
    D   oral metronidazole is useful in treatment of acute episodes
    E   peppermint oil may relieve the symptoms

18.16 A **True**   the inhaler technique should also be checked
      B **False**  vitamin K would affect warfarin-sensitive clotting
                   factors (II,VII,IX,X) for 1–2 weeks. If bleeding
                   occurred, plasma would bring the INR down without
                   compromising subsequent warfarin therapy.
                   Prednisolone could be continued
      C **False**  erythromycin potentiates warfarin and may have
                   been responsible for the prolongation of
                   prothrombin time
      D **True**   a sensible precaution
      E **False**  protamine is used to antagonise the effect of heparin

18.17 A **True**
      B **False**
      C **False**
      D **True**   Most doctors would recommend this, although there
                   is some dissent
      E **True**   both streptococcal infections and penicillin have
                   separately been implicated in causation

18.18 A **True**   the only indication for indomethacin in this patient
                   would be acute gouty arthritis, but she has no joint
                   pain
      B **False**
      C **True**   thiazides compete with uric acid for excretion in the
                   urine
      D **False**  routine prophylaxis against hypokalaemia is not
                   necessary. Only if she developed hypokalaemia
                   would intervention be necessary
      E **True**   the urea may rise because of dehydration from
                   overenthusiastic diuresis, the blood sodium and
                   potassium might decrease. Body weight (decrease) is
                   an excellent means of monitoring the treatment of
                   cardiac failure; her weight could increase after
                   indomethacin because non-steroidal anti-
                   inflammatory drugs sometimes cause salt and water
                   retention

18.19 A **False**
      B **True**   antispasmodic
      C **False**  only of use for inflammatory bowel disease
      D **False**
      E **True**

**18.20   In obtaining and distributing information about drugs**

   **A** 'yellow cards' to record adverse effects suspected to have been caused by drugs are sent to the Association of the British Pharmaceutical Industry (ABPI)

   **B** leaflets inserted in drug packages have to be approved by the drug licensing authority in Great Britain

   **C** bottles of tablets need not be labelled with the name and strength of the drug provided that the frequency of dosing is clearly shown

   **D** the Committee on Safety of Medicines writes data sheets for new drugs to be sold in Great Britain

   **E** it is important that patients should be told about swallowing tablets or capsules with food or fluid

18.20 A **False**   these are sent to the Committee on Safety of
Medicines (CSM). However, the CSM will supply lists
of side-effects reported with certain drugs but not in
relation to any specific products of any manufacturer

    B **True**   the manufacturer is legally bound to seek this
approval The Medicines Division of the DHSS is the
licensing authority but it receives advice from the
CSM

    C **False**   the bottles should be labelled for safety, 'the tablets'
or 'the capsules' is unacceptable

    D **False**   the data sheet is written by the manufacturer, but
must be approved by the Medicines Division of the
DHSS

    E **True**   if not taken with fluid some tablets stick in the
oesophagus, e.g. slow K; food decreases absorption
of some drugs like ampicillin

# Chapter 19

**19.1** **In generalised loss of hair from the scalp**
   A  cyclophosphamide could cause this
   B  minoxidil topically may promote new hair growth
   C  prednisolone could cause this
   D  regrowth of hair may occur after stopping cytotoxic therapy
   E  thyroid function tests should be performed

**19.2** **The following drugs are appropriate for treatment of the conditions mentioned**
   A  dapsone and dermatitis herpetiformis
   B  flucloxacillin for methicillin resistant staphylococcus aureus (MRSA)
   C  cis-platin for the nephrotic syndrome
   D  oestradiol plus a progestagen for male-pattern baldness
   E  captopril for heart failure

**19.3** **With regard to a 70-year-old female with osteoporosis**
   A  calcitonin will relieve bone pain
   B  the serum calcium is likely to be decreased
   C  a myopathy may occur in association with this
   D  calcium and vitamin D is sometimes given
   E  oestrogens may be of benefit

**19.4** **A 75-year-old woman is admitted with a history of confusion and falls. On admission her blood pressure was 158/88 lying and 96/58 standing. She has been taking amylobarbitone 200 mg at bedtime and imipramine 50 mg three times daily for as long as her relatives can remember. The following are correct**
   A  confusion is probably a result of severe depression and so the imipramine should be increased
   B  the amylobarbitone should be stopped immediately
   C  the imipramine should be stopped immediately
   D  both amylobarbitone and imipramine doses should be decreased gradually and eventually stopped
   E  imipramine probably caused the postural hypotension

19.1 A **True**  as may many other cytotoxics

B **True**  may be successful in male pattern baldness.
Increased hair growth is a recognised complication of
systemic treatment with minoxidil for hypertension

C **False**

D **True**  but this is not always the case

E **True**  since hypothyroidism may occasionally be a cause

19.2 A **True**  the other skin condition for which dapsone is used is
leprosy

B **False**  MRSA is resistant to all penicillinase resistant
penicillins

C **False**  cisplatin is a cytotoxic drug

D **False**

E **True**  captopril and the other available angiotensin
converting enzyme, inhibitor, enalapril are both of
value in the treatment of heart failure

19.3 A **False**  used only in Paget's disease but recent trials suggest
possible use in osteoporosis

B **False**  it is always normal as opposed to the decrease seen
in osteomalacia

C **False**  a proximal myopathy and 'waddling' gait occur with
osteomalacia

D **True**  Hypercalcaemia is a danger with vitamin D especially
in renal failure

E **True**  oestrogen decreased numbers of fractures and loss
of height when given long-term in one study. They
have disadvantageous side-effects and should not be
given without a progestagen to women who have not
had a hysterectomy. Postmenopausal osteoporosis is
a bad preventable disease — look it up

19.4 A **False**  confusion may occur as a result of depression but
here, the drugs are the most likely causes

B **False**  sudden withdrawal may cause fits

C **False**  sudden withdrawal of tricyclic antidepressants which
have been given for a long time (over 1 year) and in
high dosage can result in a withdrawal syndrome
including abdominal pain, diarrhoea, blurred vision,
salivaton, bradycardia and confusion

D **True**

E **True**  imipramine is well known to cause postural
hypotension, it depletes noradrenergic nerve endings
of noradrenaline by preventing reuptake of
noradrenaline after it has been released at nerve
endings

**19.5**  An elderly man had been taking Aldactide (combination of spironolactone and hydroflumethiazide) and Moduretic (combination of hydrochlorothiazide and amiloride) for hypertension and cardiac failure. On admission his plasma sodium was 125 mmol/l and potassium was 6.5 mmol/l. He had mild ankle oedema, no sacral oedema or third heart sound, he also had gynaecomastia. It is likely that

A   stopping Aldactide would cure his gynaecomastia
B   the plasma sodium would return to normal if the drugs were stopped
C   calcium resonium enemas should be given immediately
D   frusemide should be added to the treatment
E   his blood urea and glucose may well be raised

**19.6**  Nasal congestion may occur as a result of the following drugs

A   warfarin
B   adrenergic neurone-blocking drugs like guanethidine and debrisoquine
C   long-term use of intranasal decongestants
D   anticholinesterase inhibitors like neostigmine
E   alpha blockers

**19.7**  Antibiotics should be given prophylactically under the following circumstances

A   to prevent recurrence of rheumatic fever after streptococcal infections
B   to prevent infective episodes in patients with chronic bronchitis and frequent recurrent attacks of acute bronchitis
C   peroperatively to cover insertion of hip prostheses
D   in diabetic ketoacidosis
E   during dental extraction in patients with heart valve abnormalities

**19.8**  When prescribing an oral hypoglycaemia drug

A   chlorpropamide is the preferred hypoglycaemic in elderly patients
B   tolbutamide has a short half-life and may be used when a short action is required
C   patients should be told not to take the drugs if they have not taken adequate food or are vomiting
D   success of treatment may be assessed by measuring glycosylated haemoglobin
E   in renal failure chlorpropamide can be given

19.5  A  **True**    spironolactone causes gynaecomastia
      B  **True**    both preparations contain a thiazide and a distal
                     tubular diuretic (in addition to spironolactone and
                     amiloride triamterine is a third such agent), hence
                     reabsorption of sodium is blocked at two points, this
                     often causes hyponatraemia in the elderly. The
                     inhibition of distal sodium-potassium exchange
                     results in hyperkalaemia

      C  **False**   Ion exchange resins orally or rectally are probably
                     not needed for when the drugs are stopped the
                     electrolytes will correct themselves (as happened
                     with this patient)
      D  **False**   there is no cardiac failure. The ankle oedema is most
                     likely due to prolonged sitting
      E  **True**    side-effects of the thiazides NOT of amiloride or
                     spironolactone

19.6  A  **False**
      B  **True**
      C  **True**    nasal decongestants should be given for a few days
                     only
      D  **False**
      E  **True**

19.7  A  **True**    penicillin is used
      B  **False**   the aim is to give prompt antibiotic treatment for
                     infections, this may include giving the patient a
                     supply of antibiotics to use when the sputum
                     changes colour
      C  **True**
      D  **False**   antibiotics are only given when infection is suspected
                     and after blood and other samples is taken for culture
      E  **True**    penicillin is usually used to prevent *Streptococcus
                     viridans* endocarditis. Prophylactic antibodies are
                     also used to prevent endocarditis during genital and
                     urinary tract manipulation, including urinary
                     catheterization

19.8  A  **False**   this drug is long acting and is contraindicated in the
                     elderly and in patients with renal failure
      B  **True**    therefore useful in the elderly
      C  **True**    this is often not done and may explain some cases of
                     hypoglycaemia
      D  **True**    glycosylated haemoglobin measurement will assess
                     diabetic control during the recent past
      E  **False**   the drug is excreted largely unchanged in the urine
                     hence there is an increased risk of prolonged
                     hypoglycaemia in renal failure

**19.9    The following drugs are effective in relieving muscular spasticity**
    A    dantrolene sodium
    B    chlorpromazine
    C    L-dopa
    D    diazepam
    E    baclofen

**19.10   In hepatic encephalopathy**
    A    beta blockers should be given to correct portal hypertension
    B    lactulose should be given intravenously
    C    a high protein diet is of benefit
    D    neomycin should be given orally
    E    metronidazole should be given orally

**19.11   Methicillin-resistant *Staphylococcus aureus* (MRSA)**
    A    is usually sensitive to gentamicin
    B    should be treated whenever it is isolated from hospital inpatients
    C    is almost never pathogenic
    D    outbreaks in hospital are usually caused by failure to follow standard guidelines
    E    is more virulent than the non-resistant strain

19.9   A **True**   the direct effect on skeletal muscle and hence its lack
                    of central adverse effects is an advantage
       B **False**
       C **False**  relieves extrapyramidal rigidity, not spasticity
       D **True**   sedation is a major problem with the
                    benzodiazepines
       E **True**   sedation is also an adverse effect as is hypotonia
                    from excessive dosage

19.10  A **False**  unfortunately, even when the encephalopathy is
                    associated with portal hypertension, beta blockers
                    are of no clinical benefit
       B **False**  lactulose is given orally to empty the bowel and
                    produce an acid pH in the colon so decreasing
                    ammonia absorption by favouring ionisation to
                    ammonium ions
       C **False**  a low protein, high carbohydrate diet is needed to
                    decrease urea formation and prevent body protein
                    catabolism respectively both of which favour
                    ammonium ion production
       D **True**   in an attempt to decrease gut bacterial content
       E **True**   recently shown to be of benefit

19.11  A **False**  it is usually resistant to gentamicin
       B **False**  should only be treated when there is definite
                    evidence of pathogenicity
       C **False**  although, like other *Staphylococcus aureus* strains, it
                    is commonly merely a commensal, it does cause
                    clinical infection particularly post operatively
       D **True**   isolating and screening all patients who have been
                    hospitalised in the last 6 months on admission,
                    together with isolating all patients with positive
                    swabs and swabbing all contacts are the most
                    important steps.
       E **False**  it seems to be less virulent yet it is more virulent than
                    *Staphylococcus epidermidis*

**19.12  In the management of the terminally ill**

A   intramuscular injections of drugs are unfortunately necessary because of poor oral absorption

B   diamorphine is usually preferable to morphine because of its greater efficacy

C   both diamorphine and morphine are metabolised to active metabolites

D   the presence of renal failure prolongs the half-life of morphine

E   anticholinergic drugs may be helpful in drying up bronchial secretions

**19.13  A 69-year-old patient taking long-term dipyridamole treatment consults you. You diagnose a recurrent transient ischaemic attack. Do you**

A   increase the dose of dipyridamide to 100 mg three times daily

B   reluctantly start him on warfarin

C   start him on a beta-blocker

D   stop dipyridamole and start him on aspirin

E   add sulphinpyrazone to his treatment

**19.14  An 18-year-old girl is admitted to hospital having ingested an unknown quantity of secobarbital. She subsequently needed intermittent positive pressure ventilation (IPPV). She has a plasma sodium of 127 mmol/l, other electrolytes are normal and her urine specific gravity is 1.032 with a normal urinalysis. She has no signs of volume depletion**

A   she should be given normal saline to bring up her plasma sodium

B   she should be given an osmotic diuretic such as mannitol

C   she should be given a forced acid diuresis

D   naloxone should be given i.v.

E   she should be fluid restricted

19.12 A **False**  drugs given by mouth should be given at a dosage necessary to obtain the desired effect regardless of their bioavailability

B **False**  the two drugs have equal efficacy. The only advantage of diamophine is its greater solubility making it the drug of choice for subcutaneous administration when patients cannot tolerate oral administration

C **True**  the main metabolites are morphine 3 glucuronide and morphine 6 glucuronide. The latter is almost certainly active

D **False**  morphine is hepatically metabolised. The metabolites, however, do accumulate in renal failure

E **True**  hyoscine is useful if sedation is also required whilst atropine is free of this additional effect

19.13 A **False**  dipyridamole has not been shown to be of clinical benefit although it does have antiplatelet activity in vitro

B **False**  warfarin can be considered if effective antiplatelet therapy has failed but its value is not universally accepted

C **False**  although beta-blockers are of proven benefit in secondary prevention of myocardial infarction, they have not been shown to be of benefit in transient ischaemic attack

D **True**  aspirin is the only agent of proven value in this situation. The dosage is controversial but many authorities advise 75 mg once daily

E **False**  sulphinpyrazone, like dipyridamole, is active in vitro but does not seem to confer clinical benefit

19.14 A **False**

B **False**  mannitol is usually given to reduce cerebral oedema which would not be expected here

C **False**  forced *alkaline* diuresis would he expected to help remove drug more rapidly but in practice this is not so

D **False**  naloxone is an opiate antagonist

E **True**  the electrolyte picture suggests inappropriate ADH syndrome (hyponatraemia, concentrated urine and normal volume status). The first-line therapy of this condition is fluid restriction. Both barbiturates and IPPV may cause this syndrome

**19.15  A patient taking a thiazide diuretic chronically for hypotension**

    **A**  will have a relatively high 24-hour urinary sodium excretion

    **B**  may have a mild hypokalaemic acidosis

    **C**  may have a raised plasma bicarbonate

    **D**  may suffer loss of control of hypertension as a result of taking a non-steroidal anti-inflammatory drug concurrently

    **E**  who does not experience a diuresis may not experience a hypertensive effect

**19.16  The following statements about corticosteroids are true**

    **A**  dexamethasone and betamethasone are the most potent glucocorticoids

    **B**  fludrocortisone replacement therapy is best monitored by measuring plasma renin activity (PRA)

    **C**  dexamethasone and not prednisolone would be the corticosteroid of choice in a patient with heart failure

    **D**  prednisone is a prodrug

    **E**  corticosteroids sensitise arterioles to circulating catecholamines

**19.17  The following statements about antiarrhythmic drug treatment are true**

    **A**  a beta-blocker would be the treatment of choice in a patient with mitral valve prolapse and frequent symptomatic runs of ventricular tachycardia

    **B**  i.v. verapamil pretreatment should be given prior to medical cardioversion of atrial flutter with either disopyramide or flecainide

    **C**  amiodarone is effective in both supraventricular and ventricular dysrhythmias

    **D**  lignocaine is a class I antiarrhythmic agent because it has no effect on the duration of the action potential

    **E**  digoxin inhibits sodium, potassium ATPase within myocardial cells

19.15 A **False**   during chronic dosing the urinary sodium excretion
                    is determined purely by the dietary intake
      B **False**   hypokalaemic alkalosis
      C **True**
      D **True**    mediated via renal cyclo-oxygenase inhibition
      E **False**   the hypotensive effect is independent of the diuretic
                    effect

19.16 A **True**    there is no important difference in efficacy, however
      B **True**    PRA is a sensitive indicator of sodium balance within
                    an individual
      C **True**    drugs that cause sodium retention should be avoided
                    in heart failure
      D **True**    it is metabolised to the active drug prednisolone in
                    the liver
      E **True**    this may be one of the factors that predisposes to
                    hypertension in glucocorticoid excess

19.17 A **True**    beta-blockers would be avoided in situations where
                    their negative inotropic effect would be undesirable,
                    e.g. in patients who are haemodymanically unstable.
                    In patients with normal left ventricular function they
                    are safe and effective
      B **False**   verapamil pretreatment is necessary when
                    disopyramide is used in order to avoid a reduction in
                    the degree of AV block because of the anticholinergic
                    effect of disopyramide. Flecainide does not have this
                    effect and can safely be given alone
      C **True**    it is not, however, a first-line agent because of its
                    toxicity. It is also difficult to use because of a very
                    long half-life (several weeks) and drug interactions
                    with warfarin (potentiates), digoxin (increases
                    concentrations) and beta-blockers (potentiates
                    bradycardia)
      D **False**   class 1 agents are membrane-stabilising drugs which
                    reduce the rate of rise of the action potential during
                    depolarisation. Effects on the duration of the action
                    potential further categorise these agents into class Ia,
                    1b and 1c. Lignocaine decreases the duration of the
                    action potential hence it is a 1b agent
      E **True**

**19.18    In the treatment of chronic congestive cardiac failure**

A    a plasma sodium below 130 mmol/l implies a poor prognosis

B    thiazide diuretics are ideal because of their longer duration of action compared to loop diuretics

C    calcium antagonists are a useful addition to diuretic therapy

D    therapy with the angiotensin converting enzyme inhibitor enalapril prolongs survival

E    morphine or diamorphine is indicated in patients who do not have $CO_2$ retention

**19.19    Acetazolamide**

A    may be used in high dose for open-angle glaucoma when topical therapy has failed

B    produces a diuresis due to carbonic anhydrase activity

C    produces an alkaline urine and hence may be helpful in the treatment of aspirin poisoning

D    reduces the risk of acute mountain sickness when taken prophylactically by high altitude climbers

E    has actions similar to dichlorphenamide

**19.20    The following statements about antimicrobials are true**

A    cefoxitin is a cephalosporin with good activity against Gram negative organisms, but with poor antistaphylococcal activity

B    cefotaxime and cefuroxime are both safe in renal failure

C    metronidazole and vancomycin given orally are both effective in antibiotic associated colitis caused by *Clostridium difficile*

D    clindamycin and metronidazole both have activity against anaerobes

E    mecillinam is active against staphylococci

19.18 A **True**    the hyponatraemia is a reflection of the severity of the cardiac failure and also of the extent to which diuretics have produced volume depletion

    B **False**    the thiazides are less efficacious despite their longer duration of action

    C **False**    calcium antagonists, although vasodilators, are of unproven benefit and may be harmful because of their negative inotropic effects. Verapamil is the agent with the greatest negative inotropic action

    D **True**    recently demonstrated in a prospective placebo controlled study

    E **False**    although opiates may be of benefit in acute left ventricular failure they are not indicated in chronic heart failure

19.19 A **False**    high-dose therapy is indicated only in acute angle closure glaucoma to control pressure prior to surgery

    B **False**    carbonic anhydrase inhibition produces the diuresis (and reduced aqueous secretion)

    C **False**    it does produce an alkaline urine but also produces an acidaemia which compounds the metabolic acidosis produced by aspirin and salicylate

    D **True**

    E **True**    both drugs are carbonic anhydrase inhibitors

19.20 A **False**    it is a cephamycin with good antistaphylococcal activity

    B **True**    this advantage may, in some situations, make these drugs preferrable to gentamicin

    C **True**    metronidazole has the advantage of being considerably cheaper

    D **True**

    E **False**    it is active against many Gram-negative organisms

# Chapter 20

**20.1 Bradycardia may occur as a result of treatment with**

- A clonidine
- B pindolol
- C nifedipine
- D chlorpromazine
- E terbutaline

**20.2 The following drugs are indirectly acting sympathomimetics**

- A pilocarpine
- B isoprenaline
- C amphetamine
- D tyramine
- E bethanidine

**20.3 The following antihypertensives can be given once daily**

- A minoxidil
- B slow-release nifedipine
- C bendrofluazide
- D nadolol
- E enalapril

**20.4 Are the following statements about the coagulation of blood true or false**

- A bank plasma will correct the clotting defect induced by warfarin
- B fresh frozen plasma is necessary to correct the clotting defect associated with liver disease
- C heparin will prolong the partial thromboplastin time and the thrombin time
- D warfarin will prolong the thrombin time
- E phenindione will prolong the prothrombin time

20.1  A **True**   due to reduced central sympathetic outflow
      B **True**   although a beta-blocker, pindolol usually causes only a minimal (or no) fall in pulse rate because of pronounced partial agonism
      C **False**  usually causes a mild tachycardia due to vasodilation and reflex sympathetic stimulation
      D **False**  chlorpromazine is a weak alpha-blocker and will if anything induce a mild tachycardia
      E **False**  although a selective beta$_2$ agonist it will cause a tachycardia, particularly after high doses via a nebuliser

20.2  A **False**  cholinomimetic
      B **False**  stimulates receptors ie it is a directly acting sympathomimetic
      C **True**
      D **True**
      E **False**  indirectly acting adrenergic neurone-blocking drug

20.3  A **True**   the long biological half life of this vasodilator makes once daily administration possible
      B **False**  nifedipine has a short half-life and even in slow-release formulation must be given twice daily
      C **True**   all the thiazide diuretics can be given once daily
      D **True**   atenolol and sotalol are other beta-blockers that can be given once daily
      E **True**   to date, the only vasodilator other than minoxidil that can be given once daily

20.4  A **True**   only factors II, VII, IX and X are necessary to correct the warfarin-induced defect
      B **True**   all liver-produced factors are necessary, including factor V which is not found in plasma that was not frozen immediately after separation
      C **True**   hence when laboratory monitoring is necessary, these tests can be used
      D **True**   this measures conversion of prothrombin to thrombin common to both clotting pathways
      E **True**   phenindione has an identical effect to that of warfarin

**20.5    Therapeutic monitoring of blood, serum or plasma concentrations of**
A    digoxin is often indicated
B    amiodarone is indicated during long-term therapy
C    propranolol is often helpful
D    theophylline is often helpful
E    cyclosporin A is always indicated when given to patients after renal transplantation

**20.6    In a patient with acute severe asthma**
A    maximal inspired oxygen concentration would be safe in a patient with a normal serum bicarbonate
B    triple therapy with a $beta_2$ agonist, corticosteroid and theophylline is appropriate therapy in a patient with a pulsus paradoxus of 30 mmHg, pulse of 120/min and PEFR less than 100 l/min
C    intravenous aminophylline is contraindicated in patients who may have been taking an oral theophylline
D    inhaled steroids should be started at the same time as systemic steroids
E    sodium cromoglycate may be useful

**20.7    In a patient with chronic bronchitis and emphysema**
A    doxapram may be helpful in an episode of acute respiratory failure
B    a trial of steroids may be beneficial
C    a single evening dose of a short acting benzodiazepine may be used for night sedation even if some degree of $CO_2$ retention is present
D    mucolytics should be given during acute attacks of bronchitis
E    a normal serum bicarbonate or normal $P_{CO_2}$ would enable oxygen to be administered safely

**20.8    The rate of renal excretion of a drug is usually related to**
A    the free (not protein-bound) plasma drug concentration
B    the total plasma drug concentration
C    tubular reabsorption
D    lipid solubility of the drug
E    the volume of distribution of the drug

20.5   A **True**   digoxin is almost always given to patients with atrial
                    fibrillation when the pulse should be monitored
                    as well as the serum concentrations
       B **True**   the extremely long half-life and the toxicity of the
                    drug make monitoring during chronic dosing esential
       C **False**  it may occasionally be helpful when testing
                    compliance
       D **True**   particularly when response has not been ideal. An
                    increase in dose can then be effected only if
                    necessary hence avoiding toxicity
       E **True**   approximate therapeutic ranges in renal transplant
                    patients have now been derived and make
                    monitoring crucial

20.6   A **True**   the bicarbonate (and $pCO_2$) will be raised in patients in
                    whom high inspired oxygen concentrations would be
                    dangerous
       B **True**   such a patients must be managed very aggressively
       C **False**  in such a patient a loading dose would be
                    contraindicated, but a maintenance infusion would
                    not
       D **False**  when the acute attack is over, inhaled steroids need
                    only be started as the dose of systemic steroids is
                    reduced
       E **False**  sodium cromoglycate is a prophylactic agent and is
                    ineffective in the acute phase

20.7   A **True**   doxapram is a respiratory stimulant that can be given
                    by i.v. infusion
       B **True**   a trial of steroids would only be necessary if airways
                    obstruction was present and unresponsive to other
                    bronchodilators
       C **False**  all sedatives should be avoided
       D **False**  there is no evidence that mucolytics have any effect
       E **True**   an elevated serum bicarbonate would be present if
                    $CO_2$ retention was present

20.8   A **True**   the rate of excretion (mg/min) increases with
                    increasing drug concentration whereas the clearance
                    (ml/min) usually does not
       B **False**  the free concentration is the determinant
       C **True**   tubular secretion and tubular reabsorption are
                    important for many drugs
       D **True**   water-soluble drugs are predominantly renally
                    excreted and lipid-soluble drugs are predominantly
                    metabolised in the liver
       E **False**  the volume of distribution of the drug will influence
                    the plasma half-life but not the rate of renal excretion

**20.9**    **The following drugs are excreted largely unchanged in the urine**
   A   metformin
   B   acyclovir
   C   pindolol
   D   lithium
   E   hydralazine

**20.10**    **The following drugs may be administered once daily**
   A   digoxin
   B   propranolol
   C   gentamicin
   D   spironolactone
   E   trimethoprim

**20.11**    **The following statements about the effects of drugs on the kidney are correct**
   A   potassium retaining diuretics are aldosterone antagonists
   B   non-steroidal anti-inflammatories antagonise the effects of diuretics
   C   osmotic diuretics have an effect on excretion of water but very little effect on $Na^+$ excretion
   D   thiazides predominantly affect distal convoluted tubule function
   E   loop diuretics antagonise active $Na^+$ reabsorption in the ascending limb of the loop of Henle

**20.12**    **Acute renal failure may be caused by**
   A   amphotericin B
   B   trimethoprim
   C   sulphonamides
   D   triamterene
   E   penicillamine

**20.13**    **In patients receiving chronic haemodialysis, the following drugs will be removed during dialysis**
   A   paracetamol
   B   ethanol
   C   penicillin
   D   isoniazid
   E   hydralazine

20.9  A  **True**
      B  **True**    one of the few interactions involving acyclovir is with
                     probenecid, which reduces the renal excretion of
                     acyclovir
      C  **False**   pindolol is a lipid-soluble drug which is reabsorbed
                     from the renal tubule and is predominantly
                     hepatically metabolised
      D  **True**
      E  **False**   extensively metabolised by the liver with a very high
                     hepatic extraction ratio

20.10 A  **True**
      B  **False**   at least twice-daily administration is required
      C  **False**   in the presence of normal renal function, 8-hourly
                     dosing is appropriate
      D  **True**
      E  **False**   in the presence of normal renal function twice daily
                     dosing is necessary

20.11 A  **False**   only spironolactone is an aldosterone antagonist,
                     triamterene and amiloride are not
      B  **True**    probably by a combination of pharmacodynamic and
                     pharmacokinetic mechanisms
      C  **False**   osmotic diuretics cause a nariuresis secondarily to
                     the increased urine flow rate
      D  **True**    the main effect is on the distal tubule, although they
                     do affect the proximal tubule
      E  **False**   the active process is chloride reabsorption and
                     sodium follows passively. This is blocked by loop
                     diuretics

20.12 A  **True**    distal tubules are affected first
      B  **False**
      C  **True**    some sulphonamides or their metabolites which are
                     poorly soluble may be precipitated in the tubules
                     causing obstruction
      D  **False**   interstitial nephritis is, however, a very rare
                     association
      E  **False**   penicillamine causes the nephrotic syndrome

20.13 A  **True**
      B  **True**
      C  **True**
      D  **True**
      E  **False**   the hepatic clearance of hydralazine is very rapid
                     and, in addition, hydralazine is probably extensively
                     bound to vascular smooth muscle

**20.14** **The following drugs may cause pulmonary eosinophilia**
   A  nitrofurantoin
   B  paracetamol
   C  gold injections
   D  sulphonamides
   E  phenytoin

**20.15** **The following drugs may cause pulmonary fibrosis**
   A  busulphan
   B  nitrofurantoin
   C  methysergide
   D  ethambutol
   E  hydralazine

**20.16** **Which of the following statements are true regarding rebound hypertension after abrupt withdrawal of clonidine therapy?**
   A  it is unique to clonidine
   B  it is associated with high catecholamine concentrations
   C  it occurs only after very high doses of clonidine
   E  blood pressure can be controlled with peripheral alpha blockers
   E  coexistent therapy with angiotensin converting enzyme inhibitors increases the risk of developing the syndrome

**20.17** **Analogues of vasopressin are used to**
   A  increase uterine contractility
   B  treat nephrogenic diabetes insipidus
   C  treat the polyuria of hypercalcaemia
   D  reduce ureteric spasm during therapy with opiates
   E  treat inappropriate ADH syndrome

**20.18** **Which of the following drugs are used in immunosupression after renal transplantation**
   A  cytosine arabinoside
   B  azothiaprine
   C  cyclosporin A
   D  cyclophosphamide
   E  busulphan

20.14 A **True**
B **False**   aspirin, however, may produce pulmonary eosinohilia
C **True**
D **True**
E **False**

20.15 A **True**
B **True**
C **True**   also associated with retroperitoneal fibrosis
D **False**
E **False**

20.16 A **False**   it has also rarely been described after cessation of methyldopa therapy
B **True**   presumably related to down regulation of central alpha-receptors during chronic therapy with a central alpha-agonist
C **True**   most patients reported with this syndrome had been receiving 1200–1600 $\mu$g daily
D **True**   these drugs block the adrenergic receptors responsible for the rise in blood pressure. Clonidine itself is also effective
E **False**   coexistent beta-blockers, however, may exacerbate the situation by allowing unapposed alpha stimulation

20.17 A **False**   theoretically of value but no use in practice
B **False**   *cranial* diabetes insipidus will respond
C **False**
D **False**   again theoretically might be helpful but not used clinically. Its use in other than single doses would produce dilutional hyponatraemia
E **False**   it would exacerbate the condition

20.18 A **False**
B **Truc**   until recently this was the drug of choice
C **True**   at present the drug of choice
D **True**   when azothiaprine could not be given this was the second choice
E **False**

**20.19** **Which of the following drugs can be given via the inhaled route and is available as a pressurised aerosol, dry powder and nebuliser solution**
A  beclomethasone
B  aminophylline
C  sodium cromoglycate
D  terbutaline
E  ipratropium bromide

**20.20** **Epidemiological studies have shown**
A  above the age of 45 years, systolic BP is a better predictor of risk than diastolic BP
B  cigarette smoking status at follow up is the main determinant of prognosis in survivors of myocardial infarction who smoked before their infarct
C  thiazide diuretics are more effective than beta blockers in preventing complications of hypertension in smokers
D  beta-blockers will only reduce mortality after myocardial infraction if given within 2–3 hours of the attack
E  treatment of hypertension in the elderly does not reduce the complication rate

20.19 A **True**    recently has become available as a nebuliser solution
      B **False**    theophylline is not as effective when given via the inhaled route as would be expected. No formulations are available
      C **True**    cromoglycate was the first drug to be marketed as a dry powder preparation via a breath activated system (Spinhaler)
      D **True**
      E **False**    only available as a pressurised areosol and nebuliser solution

20.20 A **True**    Framingham study
      B **True**    several follow-up studies have noted this
      C **True**    the MRC study (which used a very high dose of bendrofluazide — 10 mg) demonstrated this surprising result
      D **False**    although the benefit seems to be greater if beta blockers are given early, late intervention studies have shown benefit
      E **False**    the stroke rate fell and the case fatality for myocardial infarction fell in the European Working Party on the treatment of hypertension in the elderly study (EWPHE)